my pet

VIRUS

JEREMY P. TARCHER/PENGUIN

a member of Penguin Group (USA) Inc.

New York

my pet

VIRUS

the true story of
a rebel without a cure

Shawn Decker

JEREMY P. TARCHER/PENGUIN
Published by the Penguin Group
Penguin Group (USA) Inc., 375 Hudson Street, New York, New York 10014, USA ·
Penguin Group (Canada), 90 Eglinton Avenue East, Suite 700, Toronto, Ontario, M4P 2Y3, Canada
(a division of Pearson Penguin Canada Inc.) · Penguin Books Ltd, 80 Strand, London WC2R 0RL,
England · Penguin Ireland, 25 St Stephen's Green, Dublin 2, Ireland (a division of Penguin Books Ltd) ·
Penguin Group (Australia), 250 Camberwell Road, Camberwell, Victoria 3124, Australia (a division of
Pearson Australia Group Pty Ltd) · Penguin Books India Pvt Ltd, 11 Community Centre, Panchsheel
Park, New Delhi – 110 017, India · Penguin Group (NZ), Cnr Airborne and Rosedale Roads,
Albany, Auckland 1310, New Zealand (a division of Pearson New Zealand Ltd) · Penguin Books
(South Africa) (Pty) Ltd, 24 Sturdee Avenue, Rosebank, Johannesburg 2196, South Africa

Penguin Books Ltd, Registered Offices: 80 Strand, London WC2R 0RL, England

The author gratefully acknowledges permission to quote from: "Blasphemous Rumours,"
words and music by Martin Gore. © 1984 EMI Music Publishing Ltd. All rights for the
U.S. and Canada controlled and administered by EMI Blackwood Music Inc. All rights
reserved. International copyright secured. Used by permission.

Most Tarcher/Penguin books are available at special quantity discounts for bulk purchase for sales
promotions, premiums, fund-raising, and educational needs. Special books or book excerpts also can
be created to fit specific needs. For details, write Penguin Group (USA) Inc. Special Markets,
375 Hudson Street, New York, NY 10014.

Library of Congress Cataloging-in-Publication Data

Decker, Shawn.
My pet virus : the true story of a rebel without a cure / Shawn Decker.
        p.   cm.
ISBN 1-58542-525-7
1. Decker, Shawn.   2. Hemophiliacs—Virginia—Biography.
3. HIV-positive persons—Virginia—Biography.   I. Title.
RC642.D43   2006   2006044620
362.196'97920092—dc22
[B]

Printed in the United States of America
1   3   5   7   9   10   8   6   4   2

Book design by Stephanie Huntwork

To all my guardian angels, both living and dead

contents

*"I don't want to start
any blasphemous rumours
but I think that God's
got a sick sense of humour
and when I die
I expect to find Him laughing."*

—DEPECHE MODE

my pet

VIRUS

when bad names
happen to good people

You probably don't know this, but most hemophiliacs hate to be referred to as hemophiliacs. It has to do with not wanting to be defined by an illness. You don't call someone with cancer a "cancerite," or someone with multiple sclerosis a "multisclerosisist," do you? Also, the word "hemophiliac" means "one who loves blood." Ask any person with a bleeding disorder whether or not they love blood and you'll probably be served a knuckle sandwich.

Personally, I don't mind being called a hemophiliac. I enjoy being confident in the knowledge that I can bleed anyone in a bar or pool hall under the table. But I'm in the minority of a minority, and as far as the severity of the condition goes, I'm somewhat of a lightweight, classified a "mild hemophiliac." That, coupled with the fact that I haven't had to deal with hemophilia on a regular basis since my bumbling childhood, softens the impact and connotation of the word for me.

Still, being pegged with a medical condition can be a real downer. My problem with the alternative lingo—"a person with hemophilia"—is that it's much too wordy. I should be able to introduce myself and my gaggle of viruses and diseases without needing a hit of oxygen. And I'm obviously a person; being required to verbalize that fact is insulting, even though it doesn't hurt to remind some doctors, who are capable of forgetting that patients are people, too. So I came up with a new word for the modern-day hemophiliac: "thinblood."

One has to be careful about labeling people; I mean, you should see what happened to the guy who started calling hemophiliacs "bleeders"—it wasn't a pretty sight. But there may be a historical precedent for "thinblood." Perhaps the true origin of the word developed somewhere in Native American culture. Isn't it entirely plausible that several thousand years ago someone walked the Earth who answered to the name of Thinblooded Bleeding Horse? Another good Indian—I mean Native American—name for someone of my ilk would be Bleeds Like Waterfall.

Stephen Gendin would have loved Bleeds Like Waterfall and thinblood. Who is Stephen? He was a friend of mine who was gay, and I'm using the past tense not because he prayed and became straight but because he passed to spirit in 2000. When Stephen was at college, someone took his favorite jacket and wrote "COCKSUCKER" on the back of it in permanent Magic Marker. Most would have shamefully discarded the garment, but Stephen proudly wore his jacket as if nothing happened. When asked about the writing on the back, he simply said, "Oh, that's my gang."

Being HIV positive kind of makes you feel like you *are* part of a gang—feared by the public, misunderstood, avoided in dark alleys. For some, this feeling can come even when being embraced, and that's why I think it is equally important that we try to change our own image, which should start not with how others view us but how we view ourselves. But we'll get to people with HIV in a minute; for now, thinbloods have some other issues to deal with.

To the blood industry, thinbloods are the canaries in the coal mine, because whenever a hip, new viral infection is out there, we get it first. I should know. I've gotten hepatitis B, HIV, and hepatitis C, all from tainted blood products.

Medical fact: a blood-product treatment is literally an orgy of plasma. Thousands of donor samples are combined, and the clotting factor that I am deficient of—factor VIII—is extracted into a concentrated form that is injected via needle. I've never received a traditional, one-donor blood transfusion, but I've had hundreds of blood-product treatments, which means I've been exposed to millions of people's blood. I guess you could say I'm a blood whore.

Thinbloods who've gotten HIV not only juggle a compromised immune system and genetic disease, they also deal with the ignorance and stigma that goes along with AIDS— the homophobia, job discrimination, dating woes, family drama, and having to receive those horrible AIDS benefit CDs as Christmas presents every December.

Many of those cursed events are out of one's control, but not the name change. And I have a feeling the switch from "hemophiliac" to "thinblood" will do us some good. Just look at Elton John, who was born Reginald Kenneth Dwight. Do you think "Reginald Dwight" could have played anywhere outside of a few dirty, roach-infested Nashville dives? Highly doubtful. So if Sir Elton can make a life-altering name change, then why not an entire community?

Which brings me back to people with HIV and AIDS.

Even within our own infectious ranks, there is a hierarchy. Those newly diagnosed with HIV are relieved that they don't have an AIDS diagnosis yet, while those with the dreaded "scarlet A" diagnosis look down their nose at the newbies— "Beginners," they scoff. Aside from bragging rights, is there really a purpose in distinguishing one from the other?

In the old days, the difference between being "HIV positive" and "having AIDS" was like the difference between swimming in the ocean with sharks and sitting in your bathtub with one. HIV was the virus that, over time, wore down the immune system and led to what are called "AIDS-defining illnesscs": Kaposi's sarcoma, lymphoma, encephalopathy, cryptococcosis, isosporiasis, and severe Tetris addiction.

These days, in countries with access to decent health care, an AIDS diagnosis doesn't necessarily mean the end. In 1987, I was diagnosed with HIV. And in 1999, I got an AIDS diagnosis, but thanks to modern medicine—and the fact that I'm American—I'm healthy enough to do pretty much what I want to do.

The colorful history of how *all* people living with HIV and AIDS have been described over the last twenty-five years has been, well . . . colored by the worst descriptions since the term "colored." I'm not sure what's more upsetting—having AIDS or having to watch people on the news talk about AIDS. In the last twenty years the media have called us "the afflicted" (cool name for a punk band, shitty title for some-one living with an illness), "terminal," "end-stager," "vic-tim," "sufferer," and (my own personal favorite) "full-blown AIDS victim." We've been dying not just from weakened immune systems and lowered T cell counts, but also from weakened self-esteem and lowered expectations. Some have tried to put a new stamp on people with AIDS, the most visi-ble of which is "PWA" (person with AIDS). But even that makes me think of "POW," and I don't like thinking of my-self as a prisoner of my pet virus.

That's why I've created another new term, one that *all* people living with HIV and AIDS can be proud of: "positoid."

And those of you out there who aren't infected, don't feel left out—you are negatoids.

As happy as "positoid" sounds, I've gotta fess up that, in my worst hours growing up with HIV, I sometimes wondered why I couldn't have been Tom Cruise instead. But just as quickly I realize I could have been Tom *Arnold*. And if I were Tom Arnold, I'd probably thank my lucky stars that I wasn't some smart-assed hemophiliac AIDS sufferer. Life is a complicated mixture of the sour and the sweet, the proof being that since I originally typed this paragraph, Tom Cruise has become a publicist's worst nightmare, while Tom Arnold and I—inexplicably—are thriving.

I can be laid-back about my lot in life because I now realize that I was destined for a life of medical drama from day one. I was born in the month of July, and my horoscope sign is a disease (Cancer). The symbol for Cancer? A crab (the sexually transmitted critter). Not only that, my parents named me Shawn Timothy Decker, which makes my initials S.T.D. and could explain my preoccupation with creating new names.

Maybe my life isn't so enviable; and, yes, I've been given a lot to deal with in my first thirty years of living. But that's the circle jerk of life: everyone has obstacles and labels to overcome, mine just involve life-threatening medical conditions. And instead of dying like I was supposed to, I became a thinblooded positoid with a sick sense of humor, merrily making my way in a thickblooded world.

life as a thinblood

Initially everything seemed good to go. My weight was normal, I ate well, and I was blessed with all my limbs when I came into this life with a whimper as, according to my mother, Barry Manilow's "Could It Be Magic" played on the radio. My mother figured she'd just scoop me up, take me home, and that my birth would be one of only a handful of times we'd be hanging out in a doctor's office. But months later, my circumcision would tell a different tale: my little fellow bled like a stuck pig.

Also known as "the royal disease" because of its prevalence in the British royal families of the eighteenth century, hemophilia is a pretty severe condition. Deficiency of factor VIII, a clotting protein, can cause severe damage in the joints and can transform minor accidents, such as getting in a fender-bender or slipping on a banana peel, into serious health hazards. The odds of being born with the genetic bleeding disorder are roughly one in ten thousand for males, and much less for females, who are the carriers of the defective gene. My ability to pull off this long shot may explain my recent fascination with gambling in Las Vegas, which thus far has not translated into chips at the roulette table.

In the eighteen months before I was officially diagnosed with hemophilia, my parents would get menacing glares whenever I was in the hospital, once again covered in bruises no one could really explain. And they weren't the only ones who got funny looks. Instead of crawling, I walked around on my hands and feet with my diaper-covered ass pointing straight up in the air. I wasn't pretending to be a puppy dog; I was on all fours because the floor hurt my knees, which turned Prince-purple every time I put my baby weight on them.

As a result of the telltale hemorrhaging, doctor after doctor informed my parents that I might not survive childhood, and John Travolta's stirring role as an immune-compromised teenager in *The Boy in the Plastic Bubble* became the model that my existence would be patterned after. "If you can just get Shawn settled into the bubble before he gets too much older," I can imagine them saying, "then he'll never know the difference." To their credit, Mom and Dad stopped short of encasing me in a plastic apparatus, but not by much.

While other toddlers played with metal Tonka trucks, I kept myself busy with foam rubber cars. After I bumped my head on a corner of the room, my mother worked on plans for a house that included no sharp edges—a literal "biodome" to keep me alive. Strict supervision and discipline were my way of life, and I was constantly being fussed over. But even though Mom and Dad were worried about hemophilia, their biggest concern for my well-being wasn't my bleeding disorder. It was my thickblooded brother.

Kip, two years older and quite brutish, was warned not to play too roughly with his fragile sibling. His incredible strength and my frailty were a combustible combination, which meant he was seldom allowed to be within ten yards of me. Poor bro; he'd hoped for a sibling but had gotten a restraining order instead. At age six, Kip became fed up with my general uselessness and put his ever-developing linguistic ability to use.

"I hope Shawn dies," he told Mom.

"Why would you say that?" she replied.

"Because," Kip said, "Shawn doesn't have a life. You and Dad don't let him do anything. He'd have more fun in Heaven."

At the time, I was in the hospital because of serious internal hemorrhaging. My liver was failing because I'd been infected with hepatitis B through the use of tainted blood products, the first in a long line of infectious diseases I would go on to collect—instead of stamps or coins like other

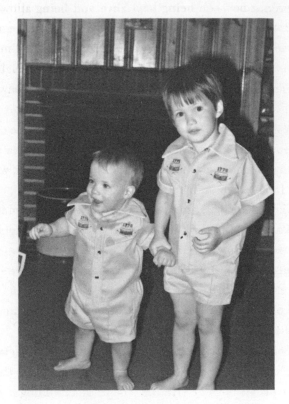

**My brother, age three,
shares his fashion sense with me.**

kids. I was in a coma for a day, and as my family waited in the hospital, Mom thought about Kip's reasoning: Was there a difference between being kept alive and being allowed to live? And considering where I was now, did all of the overly protective measures make up for everything that I'd missed out on? Ultimately, Mom and Dad decided Kip was right. "If God lets Shawn live," Mom told a doctor who was at my bedside, "then I'll let him live, too."

My brother grew to regret his influential words, because I pulled through like a champ and, as such, became a completely spoiled brat who could do whatever I wanted, whenever I wanted.

Many people feel sorry for me, but the true victim in the Decker family is Kip. When I was born his birthright was clipped off, discarded along with the crusty remains of my umbilical cord. A crucial aspect of his development—a license to pummel his younger sibling at will—was never available to him, which is just as detrimental as not knowing the difference between letters and numbers.

I'm convinced the source of the older sibling's desire to issue beatdowns comes from the innate knowledge that he has to *actually learn everything.* The younger sibling is just a parrot, gobbling up crackers without really knowing what the hell is going on. My brother could never act on his natural inclination to thrash me, until one winter's day when I was eight and he was ten.

During a snowball fight in which fate pitted brother

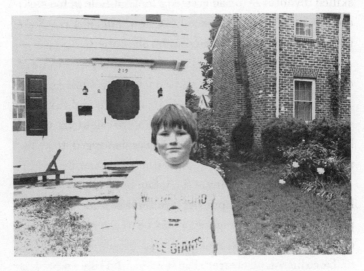

My thickblooded brother and bodyguard, Kip.

against brother on opposing teams, I stared across the lawn at Kip, separated from me by two walls of snow. Always the skilled inventor, Kip had created a lookout hole in his barricade to keep tabs on the enemy, and whenever I ran out to gather fresh snow I got pelted with snowballs.

During a lull in combat, I hatched a plan to use my dead-eye aim to plug up that spy hole, to force Kip's team of cowardly warriors to fight like men. I wound up and threw the snowball with icy precision, wedging it right in there—bull's-eye! The only hitch? That eye belonged to a bull named Kip Decker.

Kip screamed in agony at the moment of impact. I tucked behind my barricade, put my head between my knees, and prayed the way they taught you to prepare for nuclear fallout during the Cold War years.

Once his vision cleared, Kip saw red, and like a polar bear he plowed through the wall of snow that separated us, picked me up, and tossed me around like a doll, batting me to and fro with his massive paws. The best way to stave off an animal attack is to play dead, so I lifelessly lay on the ground until the ravaging was over, and I didn't move until I heard the footsteps of my burly assailant tromp off slowly in the distance . . . The extra padding of my winter layering afforded me pretty good protection, and despite the brutality of the assault, I wasn't dealt any serious damage. Not so for one of my buddies.

One day during an innocent game of Photon—the poor man's Laser Tag—Kip suspected my friend Patrick of resetting his gun, thus erasing all the hits Kip had painstakingly tallied against him. When my pal protested the claim, Kip picked him up and body-slammed him on the sidewalk, which caused the gun to reset upon impact. As Patrick writhed in pain, Kip picked up his gun, waved it in front of his glazed-over eyes, and shouted, *"See? No hits!"*

With his temper, you can see why my parents got nervous anytime Kip and I roughhoused. They'd yell, "Kip, don't hurt your brother!" But the body slams—on me, at least—were always delivered on a bed or sofa.

Midway through my kindergarten year, we moved into a neighborhood that was popular with families, thanks to its close proximity to the elementary school. Jared lived right across the street, and two doors down, there was Michael. The only thing these two guys had in common was their red hair and joint status as my best friend.

Jared had a long face and probing eyes and was wise in many matters, honing his life skills—he was the first kid I knew to find out who the Beatles were—by observing his three older brothers. Michael, a round-faced boy with a bowl cut, possessed less worldly knowledge, but had the most toys and the biggest yard. The three of us lived on Crompton Road, and soon we became known as the Crompton Road Crew.

The first thing I did when I moved onto Crompton was run down to Michael's house, where we wrestled in his front yard until I got a bloody nose. Before I arrived on Crompton, Jared and Michael had engaged in a battle of their own that ended when the impulsive Michael bit his foe square on the ass, his teeth sinking right through Jared's blue jeans, drawing blood. So if bloodshed was how Michael marked his territory, I guess I lucked out.

On the first day of first grade, before the teacher could hand out pencils, Michael discovered a box of crayons under his desk. "Hey, Shawn!" he said, and when I looked back, I saw that he'd drawn a big, round ass in black Crayola crayon on his wood-top desk. Michael's obsession with asses and his complete lack of restraint made things a lot more fun, both in school and on Crompton Road.

One afternoon my thickblooded, redheaded pals decided that the fun thing to do was to jump off Michael's garage roof. I figured I'd just wait it out until they got bored, and then join in on the next event—maybe a more thinblood-friendly game of Ms. Pac Man on Atari, some GI Joe, or we could even mash up Michael's garden, reenacting our favorite slasher flicks, *Friday the Thirteenth* and *The Children of the Corn*. (Michael's mom eventually decided that the corn would just have to come from the grocery store.)

But Michael and Jared, all jacked up on adrenaline after flying off that roof a few times, noticed that I was just standing there, which was kind of a buzzkill. When they started to encourage me to take the leap of faith as well, I declined, knowing better.

That's when they got agitated. *"Chicken!" "Bock bock!"*

The dreaded chicken taunt was so severe that I decided the only way to silence the clucking tongues was to just get it over with and jump. So I climbed up, perched unsteadily as my ankles shook below me, and took a deep breath before looking down. Suddenly my friends, no longer actin' the fool, were being supportive. "See? It's not so high! You can do it!" I swallowed my fear and dropped as gingerly as I could. When I crashed down, I knew my ankle was toast. As I gimped home like a mangy, defeated street dog, I knew the taunting wasn't quite over yet. "You did *what?*" my parents said with an our-son-is-such-a-dumbass look on their faces. "You know better than that!"

Of course I did. But my friends didn't, and it wasn't until they saw me hobbling around on crutches for two weeks that they grasped an understanding of what hemophilia did to me, and that limpin' ain't easy.

Michael and Jared got along pretty well with Kip, who enjoyed free rein when it came to protecting his little brother. "If anyone ever messes with Shawn," Mom instructed, "you kick their ass!" She considered his height and rotund shape valuable assets.

One day my bodyguard was called to duty when the Crompton Road Crew were playing an intra-neighborhood game of football with an opposing street. My friends knew of my condition, and though they refused to allow me to run touchdowns past them, dancing like Deion Sanders, they made sure not to be any rougher than necessary. But this game was different. Bragging rights were at stake, and nobody on the other team knew I was a thinblood.

After catching a pass and running for a first down, I was tackled. As I lay on the ground, about to get up, another kid felt the need to deliver an extra blow for good measure. Kip, witnessing the infraction, sensed danger and barreled in to deliver a crushing blow of his own, knocking the kid to the ground. When he got up, Kip did it again. And again. And again. Fortunately for the boy, there wasn't a sidewalk nearby.

Nothing in organized sports could compare with some of the games we invented on Crompton Road. Our favorite, Sack Ball, was a variation of Smear the Queer, the game where you throw the football in the air and try to tackle the idiot who catches it. Our version was the most dangerous play of football—the kickoff return—repeated over and over again. Somehow I avoided serious injury playing Sack Ball.

As everyone on Crompton Road learned to deal with my life as a thinblood, Kip enjoyed the prototypical existence of a thickblood. At age seven, he played on a farm league baseball team, and it wasn't long before I wanted a slice of that Americana pie for myself.

Since I was too young to join the all-star roster, I became the batboy, proudly fetching the sticks for my brother and his teammates. The next season I'd be eligible to play, but my parents hoped my attention would soon be diverted, like a few years later when I signed up for karate lessons only to quit after the first week (I really just wanted the karate gi, like the one worn by Ralph Macchio in *The Karate Kid*). But the waiting period for baseball passed as quickly as an uncle's gas at Thanksgiving, and at age six I started my own career on the field, hemophilia be damned.

Of course, there were a few risks involved.

"Never slide into base," my coach told me, fearing that I would sprain my ankle. What if a baseball was speeding toward me? "Just get out of the way," he cautioned. This all sounded very dangerous but I was more than ready for my team jersey, which, like Army-issue combat fatigues, signified there was no turning back. I wasn't worried, not a bit.

I also felt safe because the coach happened to be my father, Buddy Decker. All my friends loved him because he was the only dad who took us all to the movies, always spotting a friend if he was a few bucks short. My parents made everyone call them "Buddy" and "Pam," because, as my mom noted with slight venom, "Mrs. Decker is *Buddy's mother, Nanny!*"

Dad possessed a repertoire of off-color remarks that he used like a housewife crossing off her grocery list at Kroger, and Kip and I always had a front-row seat to his ranting and raving. Unless we were riding in the car with Mom and Dad, in which case we had a back-row seat. Like the winter morning when we were in the car, waiting for Mom to come out of the house.

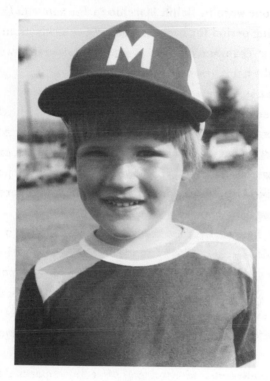

**I loved playing baseball
with my dad as the coach.**

"Goddammit," Dad said, fidgeting with his enormous glasses as he turned up the heat, which continued to blow cold air on him for his efforts. "Your mom's in a big fuckin' hurry, rushing me out of the house so I can't even take a piss, and now we're out here playing with our frozen balls . . . *Shit!*" Finally, Mom stepped out of the house, making her way to the car at a modest pace before going back to the house to make sure the door was locked. "Oh, come on already, dammit," Dad continued. "No one's stupid enough to break into a house in this weather!" As if it were wired to the door by some kind of invisible pulley system, Dad's mouth immediately closed as Mom opened the car door. As she sat down, he greeted her with a loving, "Ready to go, hon?"

My only baseball injury occurred while I was sitting on the bench in between innings. An outfielder attempting to throw the baseball to the pitcher overshot and the ball hopped and skipped until it crashed into my unsuspecting ankle. As I iced myself, I vowed to never take my eyes off of those damn thickbloods again. With blood-product treatments I didn't have to worry about my fate on or off the field, and anything that didn't kill me instantly could be taken care of with a simple injection of concentrated blood plasma.

The invention of factor VIII treatments was a lifesaver, as well as a life changer, for people like me. If a thinblooded father wanted to hop on Space Mountain and chase his kids

around Disney World, his trusty concentrate would ensure
that he could return home and not have to take off a week of
work because his knees were locked up from internal hemorrhaging. For kids the blood products meant that a normal
life—one including baseball *and* Sack Ball—was possible.

With each passing inning on the baseball field, my parents' concern subsided. All was going well, and as the kids
ran around the field aimlessly and the action played out as if
on slow-motion replay, my parents wondered why they had
been so concerned in the first place. Then the other crutch
dropped. During a game one evening, the opposing team's
pitcher was firing away at us like Dick Cheney on a duck hunt
and, one by one, he was picking us off.

My team's bench was starting to look like the waiting area
outside the emergency room, full of broken bodies and broken spirits. The cooler, packed with sodas meant to be enjoyed after the game, turned into a makeshift medical kit,
the cold six-packs used as icepacks and administered as the
casualties grew. One kid on our team cried, and he was five
players away from taking his turn at bat.

For the first time since I suited up to play ball, I was nervous, too. As coach, Dad could have thrown someone else to
the wolf in my place, but he knew that wasn't fair to the other
parents. "Just get out of the way," he said as he patted me on
the back and sent me in. True to form, the pitcher just smiled
as I dodged not only his fastest fastball but a trip to the hospital as well. Our team struck out and returned to the safety

of the outfield and infield, which meant that I was now the one pitching.

Mom had seen enough. Not the kind to mince words, Pam Decker will let you know if she's angry, and I saw her destroy many unqualified doctors and interns—clueless about hemophilia—when I was growing up. "Okay, Shawn, you know what to do," she yelled from the sidelines as I walked to the pitcher's mound.

In spots like this, it was hard being the son of Pam and Buddy Decker. In public, Mom was the bad cop and Dad was the good cop, and, in a pinch, it was always better to side with Mom because her tirades were far less comical than Dad's. But in this case, Dad was *the coach*, and I was conflicted: Do I make the boss happy at the risk of disappointing my play-by-the-rules dad?

As I stood perched like a sniper, I walked player after player, throwing the ball just out of swinging range, as I waited for the pitcher's turn to bat. The game was close, but the stakes were much higher than winning and losing; if my team was going to be in any shape to continue the season, the carnage needed to end. When the pitcher stepped up to the plate, the bases were loaded. A hit would ensure victory, and as he dug his heals into the dirt and rocked back and forth, waiting for the pitch, I wound up, leaned back, and threw the ball as hard as I possibly could. Expecting the wide shot that had walked his teammates, he'd leaned right into my pitch.

The ball slammed into his wrist and he burst into tears, screaming, "Ohhhhhhh! Ohhhhhhhh! Ohhhhhhhhhhh!" Mom cheered raucously from the sidelines, leaping up from her folding chair to give her son the standing ovation usually reserved for school chorus performances and flawless report cards.

Though all the parents on our side were just as happy, they were much less animated in their glee. One person who didn't join in the celebration was my dad, who didn't seem pleased. He came to the mound and threatened to take me out of the game. Eventually the game ended, and as usual, Dad made sure all of his players had a ride home. As we were safely out of earshot, he leaned down, put his arm around me, and whispered in my ear, "I'm so glad you hit that little motherfucker."

Sociopathic baseball players aside, the root of my thin-blooded anxiety wasn't too hard to locate, as it was literally right under my nose: nosebleeds, to be exact. They could be trickle-down economics one week and full-blown recessions the next, and when they were less complicated, I merely held my head back with a cold, damp cloth on my neck and a trusty box of tissues by my side. If that didn't work, there was always the liquid syrup, Amicar, which tasted like a bottle of Boone's Farm mixed with a shot of tequila. It was nasty stuff, and only worked on mild bleeds.

When I was four I was exposed to hepatitis B after being

treated, and from that point on Mom, who was in charge of my medical care, did everything possible before resorting to blood-product treatments. If we couldn't handle a nose-bleed at home, Mom called in our ENT (ear, nose, and throat) doctor, Ron Fischer.

Dr. Ron enjoyed scooting around in his rolling chair while humming along to the Muzak that constantly echoed through his office. The place was adorned with medical charts and graphic depictions of what the inside of one's ear really looks like. Pictures of his family as well as his patients, including one of me in my baseball jersey and cap, covered the walls. Every time I showed up, the ladies of the office would run up and hug me, which made visiting Dr. Ron just like visiting one of my friends on the block, minus the bloodshed.

While my other playmates owned an impressive arsenal of the latest toys, Dr. Ron gave me access to what could best be described as medieval torture devices. To drain my nose and get a proper look at a bleed, he used a machine that acted as a suction device, and though it never actually caused pain, I sometimes worried that parts of my brain were being sucked out through that tube. To this day I panic whenever someone fires up a vacuum cleaner.

After clearing the way, Dr. Ron would get a good look up my nostril, which he gently pried open with tongs. Once he located the source of the bleed, he'd pack the tender area with cotton dipped in a blue numbing solution. The "blue-berry cotton candy" was in preparation for cauterization involving the use of silver nitrate sticks, about six inches in length, which were stuck up my nose to burn the skin closed. Thank God for numbing solution.

With the aid of his metal gear, Dr. Ron did his best to manage my nosebleeds, but often the damage was too severe and I would have to receive a blood-product treatment. The problem thinbloods have with the blood supply is that one treatment is the equivalent of having hundreds of blood transfusions at one time, and in view of the emergence of HIV in the early 1980s, it's been said that getting a treatment before 1986 was as risky as having unprotected sex with thousands of people at once, but with none of the fun.

Even after the hepatitis B outbreak, a lot of doctors encouraged their patients to "factor up" before partaking in any type of physically straining activity, and severe thinbloods really had no choice in the matter. But Dr. Ron was skeptical of the blood industry, and though he considered blood products a great resource, they were only viewed as a last line of defense.

Though the bleeding episodes could be terribly frustrating, I never really imagined my life without them and the interesting medical procedures that followed, which gave me a chance to see a different world and meet a different group of friends. Also, I learned not to feel sorry for myself, as Mom always made me aware of the patients who had it worse than I did. "Shawn, don't complain," she said in between games of tic-tac-toe. "The person a few rooms over may be taking a dirt nap tonight."

By age ten, when I was already hip to the bleeding routine, I was approached about the possibility of not having nosebleeds—my main dilemma as a thinblood—anymore.

The technique involved sliding back the skin on the inside of my nostril in the area that was most prone to bleeding, thus creating pressure on the veins and cartilage, which would help to "naturally" stop potential bleeds before they got out of hand. My parents were sold on the idea, and when I found out that Dr. Ron would be performing the procedure, I signed up for the nose job without hesitation.

Though there were some risks, the surgery went off without any major complications, and when I came to, I saw my favorite nurse, Gail Johnson.

Over the years, Gail and I logged many late-night hours. She'd earned my respect and love with her warm personality and warmer hugs, coupled with the fact that she never missed a vein (*very* important for a thinblood). As Gail held my hand, I awoke, my nose bandaged up, and drunkenly muttered, "I'm cured," before curling up and drifting back into my anesthetic haze.

Fewer nosebleeds meant fewer trips to Dr. Ron's and the ER, and for the better part of two years, hospitals were no longer a regular part of my life. I adjusted to the thick-blooded way of life, and unhindered by the restrictions of disease, I walked blissfully forward into the great unknown, unaware that I was already living with a virus that would more than pick up hemophilia's slack.

waynesboro:
the land that time forgot

It was 1985: Madonna got married to Sean Penn, New Coke was invented and destroyed, and my fifth-grade classroom was abuzz about a new student who was joining our ranks. But before that happened there were a few things we needed to know. "Your new classmate, Frank, is here," Mrs. Warhammer said. "He's waiting in the hall because I wanted to talk to you before I introduced him. Frank is, well, he's a little bit . . . different."

My first thought was that Frank was paralyzed from the waist down, which meant he'd be in no position to challenge my kickball supremacy.

"Now, Frank doesn't look like you," she continued. "So please don't stare when he walks in."

Maybe Frank was retarded? Travis, a friend of the family, had Down's syndrome, and I saw him every six months or so. He didn't look *that* different, and we got along pretty well despite the fact that he stole my big green ten-gallon cowboy hat. Not that I'd hold Travis's crime against Frank—I'd just keep an eye on my cubbyhole whenever the new kid was around.

"You're going to meet Frank soon, but you should know that his legs are shorter than normal, and his skin is darker than yours—except for you, Billy." (Billy was the only black kid in the class.)

So Frank wasn't paralyzed. He had a tan but he wasn't black. I wondered if I would be safe sharing a classroom with this creature that was about to enter. The doorknob turned, and the door began to creak open slowly . . .

As he entered the room, not a pair of eyes left Frank Sanchez's body. And much to my dismay, his legs were not the size of his forearms, as I'd expected. They were fully functional and covered in blue jeans remarkably similar to those I was wearing. As Frank stood beside Mrs. Warhammer at the front of the class, she explained: "Frank is Mexican." I couldn't figure why she was making such the big friggin' deal over this kid.

Amigo, welcome to my hometown of Waynesboro, Virginia.

The only thing that separated Frank from the rest of the class was his ability to make paper frogs and walk on his hands.

And one day as I was trying in vain to construct a paper frog, a note landed on my desk. Curious, I unfolded the piece of paper. It was a questionnaire, posing one simple query: "Are you horny?" It was from Jared, whose brothers told him a lot about sex, bragging about their high school conquests.

I was no novice myself. My parents were pretty liberal when it came to what I could see on TV, and the first movie my dad rented when we bought a VCR was *Fast Times at Ridgemont High*. Plus, the Crompton Road Crew idolized Van Halen, mainly because of the "Hot for Teacher" video, still an all-time great.

"No," I wrote back. Then Mrs. Warhammer intercepted the note. She read the exchange and called us to her desk.

"Do you know what *this word* means?"

"No," I said, covering my tracks. "I heard it on TV one night." Jared followed my lead, pleading ignorance as well. This put all the pressure back on the adult, Mrs. Warhammer, whose mind whipped around for a couple of seconds in an attempt to find a dignified way to end the discussion. All she could come up with was: "It means *you want to have sex!*"

I'm not sure what the rest of the class—or the teacher next door—thought when they heard this outburst, but I know that our physical education teacher, Mrs. Mack, was definitely not amused by our hijinks.

Many of us had considered her hot, but not anymore: Mrs. Mack was seven months pregnant. Not only was she knocked up, she now had the unenviable task of dipping our collective toes into the waters (and other fluids) of reproductive health—yes, sex education.

She noted the differences between the male and female sex organs and warned the young ladies of their impending menstrual cycles, and we were encouraged to submit questions anonymously to her, a thoughtful move meant to protect our feelings and encourage open discussion. Mrs. Mack dutifully unfolded the questions and answered them, but would soon find that teaching dodgeball and dodging hardball questions are two entirely different fields of expertise altogether.

After patiently explaining why the penis doesn't accidentally urinate in the vagina during sex, one note was met with a cold silence. Suddenly she darted out of the room and ran down the hallway as the door closed behind her. Mrs. Warhammer wasn't in the room, so the classroom broke out into chaos. One student claimed that Mrs. Mack was crying as she exited, and fingers were pointed at me and Jared.

For once we weren't guilty. The offender was actually the nerdiest kid in class, and his question was one that is usually reserved for Hollywood's elite on the Howard Stern show. He wrote: "Have you ever had anal sex?"

Since that day twenty years ago, many a newsmagazine program has discussed how the modern-day media have given kids the fast track to adulthood via a multitude of sexually explicit programs and images. If they are even more

advanced now, can you imagine the kind of questions the little bastards are unloading on their teachers in Waynesboro
today?

My problem with the whole "new age" of sexual discovery
through television and the Internet isn't that it may be causing the youth to slut it up at an earlier age; it's that the time-
honored and sacred tradition of the porno scavenger hunt is
being rendered obsolete. When I was a kid we had to work to
see some action, and maybe I'm wrong, but unlocking the
greatest mystery of human existence should require some
guile to find the key. Plus, perhaps there wouldn't be an epidemic of overweight children if the kids had to work a little
harder for their porn.

The Crompton Road Crew's first sexual misadventure
didn't occur in Mrs. Warhammer's classroom. A few months
earlier, Michael, Jared, and I were hanging out at the local
drugstore down the street, the place where we'd buy candy
and look at the books and toys. Sometimes we'd come up
with creative names for the elderly people who patronized
the store, silly things like "Dick-nose Debbie" and "Horrible Harry the Ham Biscuit Eater."

One day, we noticed a special magazine rack behind the
counter. You could actually reach it if you got on your knees
and poked your arm around the rotating sunglasses display.
We'd slyly open a magazine and take turns trying on sunglasses as we snuck a peak. For Michael, the temptation
proved too much, and he snagged a copy of *Penthouse* and

fled the store's side-door exit in a frenzy. Jared and I followed, and soon the three of us were hiding under a tree, checking out the mind-blowing contents before stashing the rag in a bush.

The drugstore owner—who didn't press charges but did cease to sell pornographic materials—saw the crime and called our parents, who were waiting for us on the sidewalk as we slowly shuffled our feet toward them. "My parents are going to kill me," Jared sniffled, awaiting the full wrath of Catholic justice. Michael's adoptive parents likely lost a week's worth of sleep over the incident and grounded him. Me? I just got laughed at. With hemophilia, my parents didn't get too worked up over little things like misdemeanors.

By now you've probably guessed that the topic of sex wasn't taboo in my household. The Deckers enjoyed watching the *Porky's* trilogy, which detailed the adventures of Pee Wee (the guy with the little dick) and Meat (the guy with the . . . well, you get the point). *Porky's* was Dad's favorite, and it provided Kip and me with a unique opportunity to examine human sexuality. For starters, we learned that it was wise not to stick one's penis through a hole in the wall, because you never know who's going to be tugging at it on the other side.

The only time my parents put their foot down at the movie theater was when my brother and I lobbied to see

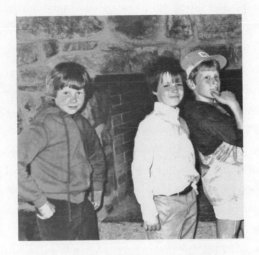

Here comes trouble: the Crompton
Road Crew—Michael, me, and Jared.

Spring Break, and even that decision wasn't based on the R rating or the T&A factor. It had more to do with Mom and Dad having already made a cinematic choice that ran a good two hours longer than *Spring Break.* I protested, but Mom promised me that someone would die in her movie, so Kip and I joined them to see *Gandhi.*

Our house on Crompton Road had two small apartments attached to it, with one room and one bathroom in each. Since my dad had a big heart, these were usually rented out to people who were in between permanent living spaces, and when Kip noticed that one of the rooms next door had been empty for a while, he lobbied for the space. About to enter his teenage years, the Kipper was ready for a little more freedom. Or he just wanted somewhere to tug it.

Now, allowing a twelve-year-old like Kip that kind of privacy might seem like a bad idea, but the chance to put a little physical distance between a plasmatically challenged little brother and a short-tempered behemoth proved irresistible, and my parents quickly caved in to Kip's demands. This move wouldn't just be one small step for Kip Decker; it would also be one giant leap for the Crompton Road Crew.

The summer day is Etch A Sketched in my mind, though the unicorns and dancing leprechauns are likely a figment of my revisionism. All the parents were hard at work, putting in the long hours necessary to feed, clothe, and house their respective families. While hanging out at my house, Jared focused his well-trained eye on something in the coat closet. I got a chair and climbed up for a closer look: it was a porno movie!

The graphic pictures on the box should have been enough, but our curiosity was far from satiated. We opened it up only to find a roll of film; this wasn't VHS, it was reel-to-reel. Michael started to giggle and let his opinion be known. *"Let's watch it!"*

Jared and I were worried. Michael, the loose cannon with the sticky fingers, really blew it for us last time with the *Penthouse* heist. My uncle was still calling me Jesse James, and if this fell through, I'd never hear the end of it. Jared's concerns were more legit; one more strike and he could be excommunicated from the Catholic Church. The Crompton Road Crew needed an expert, and I knew just who to call.

My brother possessed a knack for solving complicated and somewhat tedious problems. He'd sit in the front yard for hours trying to make a slingshot out of chopsticks and rubber bands, even if there was a store-bought model well within his grasp. If anyone could figure out how to fire this thing up, it was him. With my posse in tow, I knocked on Kip's door.

"What do you want?"

Jared held up our find and my brother's eyes lit up.

"All right, come in."

In a rare moment of sibling cooperation harking back to the Smothers and the Wrights, Kip and I inspected the film. His living quarters became our makeshift base of operations, and our team began the prolonged process of making this movie—*this mission*—work. "Go get the projector and report back," Kip said.

It was only three hours until our parents got home, so we needed to work fast. Opening the projector's metallic case was the equivalent of solving the riddle of the Sphinx. Finally, someone stumbled upon the latch, and we removed the machine slowly. Carefully. As if it were a ticking time bomb. It took close to an hour—a good fifty-seven minutes beyond most of our attention spans—but we finally hooked it up. For a movie screen, we took down one of Kip's Twisted Sister posters, turning it around to reveal the plain white side. With his windows covered and one man positioned on lookout duty, there was no way the Crompton Road Crew could fail this time.

On the very first attempt, the projector crackled to life. We couldn't figure out how to get any sound, but that wasn't a problem since we needed our ears to listen for meddling parents, who tend to pop up when least expected. As the first image of a fully clothed female emerged on the screen, our junior team of Navy SEALs let out a victory cry, and high-fives were exchanged as soon we were sharing our first glimpses of the very act that brought us into this world.

A Tony Danza look-alike appeared, but *Who's the Boss?* never provided this kind of action. As the clunky sound of the spinning reel filled the room, we watched Tony go to work on his voluptuous redheaded companion. "Is he in pain?" Michael asked as Tony grimaced. No one answered, because no one knew for sure. The two bodies pulsated in a rhythmic dance, engaging in one compromising position after another. Then it happened: the money shot. "Whoa!" One of our friends—infamous for his queasy stomach—had tagged along that day, and unable to handle the radical concept of ejaculation, he ran outside and threw up—a symbolic purging of our abandoned innocence, I guess.

failing the aids test

In the early 1980s, the initial high-risk groups for HIV infection in the United States were gay men, IV drug users, and thinbloods. Rural Americans assumed that AIDS was a big-city problem, and my hometown of Waynesboro was no different. Mom and Dad kept tabs on AIDS, but they didn't get me tested because no HIV test results meant that their wishful thinking could remain afloat.

But with each news story—a daily event in the mid-eighties—they were reminded of the predicament that I was likely in. One evening the family was watching Ted Koppel on the news giving a report on the high-risk groups for AIDS. When Kip saw hemophiliacs listed, he turned to me, pointed, and laughed. *"Ha ha! That's you!"* Of course, Kip didn't know what AIDS was, or how true his words rang. The eleven-year-old merely jumped at an opportunity to taunt his little brother. But Mom and Dad knew, and they snapped at him. "Shut up, Kip!"

When I was nine, I broke out in shingles, a chicken pox–like illness that usually affects rooftops and the elderly, as well as those with compromised immune systems. This meant trouble, so my parents took me to North Carolina to get an "unofficial AIDS test," the logistics of which I can't really explain. Somehow my immune system's strength was tested, and all I know is that the result wasn't what my parents wanted to hear. They kept the results, which weren't on the record, quiet.

Two years later I was in the sixth grade, a successful social year in which, on a dare from a friend, I managed to peck a girlfriend on the lips.

I should have been racing to school every day, but I was missing more days than all of my classmates combined. I'd get strep throat, and it never seemed to fully go away. Then an ear infection. All of which caused me to miss a few days here and there. In the spring, the school sent a letter to my parents, demanding an explanation for all of my absences.

This time, my parents got me officially tested. For three years they'd cringed every time the news came on detailing the horrors of not just living with AIDS, but dying from AIDS, and they couldn't shake the picture of their own son lying in a hospital bed, wasting away. When the test came back positive, they weren't all that surprised, but devastated nonetheless. Mom and Dad braced themselves for an uphill medical battle, but unlike with hemophilia, which we'd all learned to live with, they weren't at all confident about my chances of survival.

The State Health Department was required to contact the school and notify them of the test result, so Mom decided to confide in my sixth-grade teacher and paid her a visit one Sunday evening. Sympathetic, but also concerned about the well-being of my classmates, my teacher asked if she could speak to her doctor. Mom agreed that it was a good idea, hopeful that any irrational fears would be put to rest.

The doctor flipped out.

In 1987, people were so fearful of widespread HIV transmission that everything from handshakes to sharing number 2 pencils was suspect. The doctor had his own concerns, and revealed my HIV status to the school board and superintendent. Oh, and the doc wasn't just any small-town physician—he was the mayor of Waynesboro.

The day after my mom visited my teacher, I was sitting in class, working on an assignment, when a voice came over the intercom. *"Shawn Decker, please report to the office immediately."* My teacher made sure I took all of my belongings, and I sat on the bench where one normally awaits a dreaded meeting with the principal. I tried to think of something I'd done wrong but couldn't come up with anything. When Mom arrived, I was teary-eyed. "I know you didn't do anything," she said. "We're going home."

And that was my last day of elementary school.

Mom called the mayor, who proposed that a committee meeting be scheduled that summer—a trial of sorts—to discuss the possibility of my returning to public school. If she succeeded in swaying them, this would go a long way toward determining whether or not I'd be allowed back in. Nothing was promised, but one thing was crystal clear: AIDS *wasn't* going to be like hemophilia.

This medical condition came with tons of social issues and misunderstandings: whispers in church pews and school, parents who stopped calling and wouldn't allow their kids to come over anymore, and just a complete aura of panicked concern. People didn't understand how HIV was transmitted and felt that, when it came to a positoid, it was better to be safe than sorry. And safe, for some, meant stay the hell away—or, in the mayor's case, keep *me* the hell away.

But the mayor and Waynesboro weren't alone.

That same year a family in our same situation—the Rays in Florida—had their home burned down. A year before, an initiative in California to quarantine all people living with AIDS was proposed, and a major airline not only banned people with HIV from traveling but also recommended that anyone attempting to do so should be removed by any means necessary. So in the grand scheme of things, it would have been strange if nothing happened once the school found out I was HIV positive.

But even by 1987 standards, my parents couldn't have been prepared for the abandonment by my godparents, which, in retrospect, should have been as obvious as shingles.

My godparents were just the fun friends my parents drank beer with a few times a year while Kip and I played games with their kids. In one of the kids' rooms there was a Clint Eastwood poster on the wall, only the word "Dirty" had been taped over. "Mom made me do it," our friend said. Having the *Dirty Harry* poster was troubling to the fundamentalist Christians, but having someone with AIDS in their home was even worse, and there wasn't enough tape in the house to get around that one. They were afraid that I'd transmit my pet virus to their children, and as a result the relationship was strained. Not only that, in some churches AIDS was viewed as God's punishment for the gay lifestyle.

I don't really remember the day I was told I had AIDS, just that I was thrilled a month or so later when I was demoted to HIV. Mom explained the difference: HIV was the virus that, over time, can wear down the immune system and lead to AIDS. Even so, to my ears, "HIV" didn't sound as scary as "AIDS," and when I found out I was *just* HIV positive, I figured that gave me a few more years to live.

One of the casualties of my becoming a positoid was the Crompton Road Crew. Already a nervous nelly, Michael's mom couldn't shake the visions of her son playing with a kid with AIDS. Could any of my nosebleeds infect him? And Jared's family were even more cautious; I wasn't allowed to see him anymore, though the blow was softened when his dad got a job out of town and the family moved. All of those elements combined meant one thing: it was the end of the road for the Crompton Road Crew.

Though I was not allowed back into class, I really wanted to go on the class field trip that my parents had agreed to chaperone. But the school said no and wouldn't budge. Mom was losing her patience, and when she heard about a proposed elementary school graduation ceremony, she informed officials that we *would* be attending this event.

Dressed in a tie, button-down white dress shirt, and khaki pants, I was going to be the best-dressed kid there. Once we arrived, however, there was a last-minute change in plans. My classmates were waiting in a room, but I wasn't allowed to go in. When they filed down the hallway, I was to cut in line and go into the cafeteria with them, where the festivities were taking place. As my parents and I waited in the empty hallway, my friends found out that I was there and, one by one, they asked to go use the bathroom so they could visit me. "Shawn! Where have you been?"

My grandmother cried through the whole thing, and after I graduated from elementary school, the Deckers were asked to leave the premises because, in Waynesboro's world, AIDS—and I suppose myself as well—was not welcome.

Mom provided a good answer for any question I had about AIDS: I could get married someday. I could have kids through adoption. The way she spun it—as any good parent would—a normal adulthood was waiting, though we weren't sure if I'd make it there.

Since I've always been vain about my looks, my biggest fear was that I would look like one of those AIDS patients on the television, and more than anything else, I didn't want to end up blotchy and shriveled. With all my trips to the emergency room and my love of Rocky movies, I'd never seen anything as grim or brutal as AIDS. I decided that whatever was going to happen would happen, as I held no sway in the progression of the virus. And if things got *too* bad, I could always off myself, maybe by rotting my teeth out with excessive candy intake, or by taking a jump off of the roof of Michael's garage.

Mom prepared for the committee meeting orchestrated by the mayor that would determine whether or not I'd get back in school, and she approached this with the same ferocity Rocky brought to his training for his bout with Dolph Lundgren on steroids, stopping short of climbing a mountain in Siberia. When the day arrived, Mom was ready to teach the Waynesboro school officials about HIV/AIDS: the risk factors for transmission and, more important in our case, how the virus *cannot* be transmitted. To better her odds, she enlisted the services of my old team: Nurse Gail and Dr. Ron, and even my kindergarten teacher, who spoke as a character witness. They answered questions like "What if Shawn spits on someone?" "What if Shawn bleeds directly into someone's eye?" "What if Shawn bleeds directly into someone's mouth?"

The meeting lasted four hours, and despite her dogged determination, my mother still wasn't sure if any of their efforts and reasoning were going to make a difference one way or the other.

Afterward, Mom and Dad waited for the conclusion of the panel's thirty-minute deliberation, and the news came back: "They voted unanimously. Shawn *should* be allowed to attend school." *Victory! Victory! Victory!* But before the champagne was uncorked and poured all over the bikini-clad hos, there was one little caveat. "This isn't the final word," they said. "It's only a recommendation that goes on to the superintendent and the school board. They make the call."

But the deadline for that decision came and went, and with one week left before the start of junior high school, there was still no word on whether I was going to be allowed in. To get the scoop, Mom phoned the super, but he remained tight-lipped and elusive. That's when my father, sick to his stomach about the copious amounts of bullshit he'd been fed that summer, contacted a lawyer.

The man was a friend who once sat on the board of the Bureau of Alcohol Beverage Control, where my dad worked as a "beer cop," making sure bars and restaurants had their liquor licenses, staging the occasional raid of a drunken teen party, and, in some cases, offering a ride to jail for the town drunks, whom my dad knew on a first-name basis.

This former coworker was now practicing law with a big firm in Richmond, Virginia. Upon hearing of our plight, the lawyer contacted the Waynesboro city manager to play some hardball. His law firm represented the city, he reminded them, but they were prepared to drop Waynesboro as a client in order to take up our case against the school board for wrongful expulsion based on a medical condition. A few days later, the school board's attorney called Mom. "Now, Pam, calm down. There's no need to be bringing in any outsiders."

Well, no outsiders on *our* side, at least.

Paranoid about the lack of information, Mom used spies to keep tabs on the mayor and the superintendent's where-abouts. When she got a call from a friend informing her that there was a suspicious-looking vehicle parked in the super's backyard, Mom and Dad drove across town to the ritzy side of Waynesboro to investigate. They pulled into the alley behind the super's house, and Mom stood on the hood of her car and peered over a fence: sure enough, there was a limo. Dad noted the license plate, NUMBER1, and went home to call a fellow agent who ran the tag. "Buddy, that's the governor's car! Where did you see it?" "Oh, never mind. Thanks for checking."

Even though my dad realized that, for once, he wasn't going to get anywhere playing by the rules, it looked like he and Mom were outmanned.

But my dear old grandmother worked in the cafeteria of the junior high school we were trying so hard to get into, and one of her lunch-lady friends called from a school across town where a secret meeting was taking place. By eavesdropping, Grandmother's spy in the white hair net overheard good news: the attorney for the public school system said something to the effect of "Now, you know Pam Decker is a bitch, and we'd be better off not to piss her off anymore. So let's let the kid in tomorrow."

School was a go!

On the first day of seventh grade, Mom and I pulled into the parking lot. "Do you want me to walk you in, Shawn?" she asked. I didn't notice the police cars, and was unaware of a lot of the drama, so not wanting to be labeled a major pussy on the first day of junior high school, I refused the offer and made it in without incident.

In homeroom, an acquaintance leaned over to get my attention, and when I turned, he pointed down at my feet. "Put your socks down." They were stretched up ridiculously high, but I had no idea what he was talking about. "Fix your socks," he implored, pushing his down so they scrunched around at his ankle. "Like this." I thought he was messing with me, but then I noticed everyone else's socks were the same as his, so I followed suit.

Then came the flyer, a notice stating that a student at school was infected with the AIDS virus. Passed out to every student in the school system up to high school, it discussed the connection between hemophilia and HIV. In a kinder world, I reckon, that flyer would have been a crash course in sock-wearing etiquette.

From that moment on, I assumed that everyone knew it was me. I was the only thinblood at school, so who else could it possibly be? With all the parents gossiping and freaking out, this flyer seemed to be baiting kids into doing the same thing, and by opening up my most private secret for public consumption and scrutiny, it forced me to go into a defensive posture when it came to my virus. I was also scared and upset, because I was doing a fine job of ignoring my HIV status until I read all about it in homeroom. As futile as it seemed, I decided from the get-go that I'd guard what was left of my anonymity, and chose never to speak of HIV—not with my doctor, my closest friends, or even my brother. The resolve I made that day lasted ten years, eight years longer than doctors thought I'd live.

After lunch my guidance counselor showed me which bathroom stall to use, in case I had a nosebleed or something. Oh, and I wasn't going to be allowed in physical education class, either. I knew kids were talking as if I were an episode of *Unsolved Mysteries*, Waynesboro's answer to the Loch Ness Monster and Bigfoot. Needless to say, I was wiped out when I got home.

That year, Nessie and the Sasquatch were spotted more than I was, and I missed over a hundred days of school. But not because I was getting sick; I was pretending to be sick. So my parents went to work, worried that I was home ailing when really I was just watching my favorite soap opera, *Days of Our Lives.*

It sounds absurd, but seeing those characters endure their miserable existences not only gave my grandmother and me something to dish about, it also made me feel better about my own situation, which paled in comparison to the story lines presented on daytime television. Even on the day when, during math class, a student behind me kept saying, "I know you have AIDS." He kept at it, but I wouldn't challenge his assertion, since that would force me to talk about AIDS. Finally, a student beside me had heard enough. "So fucking what if he does?"

The bad thing was, I was right: people were talking. The good thing was that my defender probably wasn't alone, and outside of that experience I wasn't really picked on over the rumor that I had AIDS. Still, the fact that it existed was one of the reasons I'd give a little cough here and there in the mornings to stay home from school, so I could go back to bed, and wake up just in time for *Days.*

ric flair & me

I believe that America's favorite pastime may be base-ball, but America's favorite good time is professional wrestling. The outlandish outfits, the thumping entrance music, the excessive use of fireworks; it's no wonder why conservatives love the sport so much. Every day is like the Fourth of July.

Not a sport, you say? Well, let's do a comparative study. Everyone agrees that Lance Armstrong is the quintessential athlete. The guy has won numerous Tour de France titles and overcame cancer to do it. Hell, he even scored with Sheryl Crow—not many bicycle geeks could have pulled *that* off. But how long do you think Lance would last in the ring with the six-foot-seven, 320-pound Undertaker? Sure, Armstrong is resilient and has amazing stamina, but eventually the Undertaker would catch up to him and administer "The Last Ride," a potent body slam in which the 'Taker's hapless foe is hoisted high into the air before being driven down to the mat. Now *that* move takes some serious strength and skill.

I know, *but wrestling isn't real.* Well, I would argue that in terms of danger to the athletes, only one sport could possibly surpass pro wrestling in fatalities and career-ending injuries: competitive cheerleading.

Say what you will, but nothing else combines Method acting with the grace of figure skating, or fuses the emotional content of daytime television with the bare-knuckled justice of hockey. Add some crazy characters who would not be out of place in *The Wizard of Oz* and you have the perfect form of entertainment—affordable Broadway for the lower-middle class. Even more so than *Days of Our Lives*, it was in the strange world of professional wrestling and suspended disbelief that a scared kid with a life-threatening illness found an escape from AIDS. And a hero.

While most kids idolized Joe Montana and Michael Jordan, my bedroom wall was a shrine to the stars of the World Wrestling Federation (WWF) and its rival, the National Wrestling Alliance (NWA). In the WWF, the all-American Hulk Hogan ruled the land, defending his title against any evil challenger who dared to oppose his unwavering view of right and wrong. The perennial role model, Hogan captured the public's imagination and thus became the first crossover star from the world of wrestling, appearing in movies and television ads for shaving creams. After his matches, the Hulkster generously posed for his fans, giving them ample time to snap keepsake photos of his impressive biceps, his "twenty-four-inch pythons!"

Over in the NWA, Ric Flair reigned supreme. The antithesis of Hogan, Flair held on to his title by any means necessary, and though his hair was bleached to a dangerous level of blond, his nickname was "the Nature Boy." He wasn't interested in relating to the common man and often boasted of being "a jet-flyin', limousine-ridin' son of a gun." As Hulk Hogan made people feel good about themselves over in the WWF, Ric Flair made a living by pointing out that he was more than a few rungs up the social ladder. Instead of celebrating with the fans after a victory, Ric Flair hurled insults at the blue-collar fans who spent their hard-earned money to see him wrestle. "I'll take your lady home and show her what a *real* man can do!"

I loved Ric Flair. I hated Hulk Hogan. And one of my longest-lasting friendships was spawned via a mutual admiration for professional wrestling.

Mark and I were the same age, but somehow we never made it into the same classroom. While Jared's parents freaked out when I tested positive, forbidding my friend to see me, Mark's mom was a nurse, and the fact that I'd tested positive for HIV didn't faze her. When we moved off Crompton Road and closer to my new best friend, I was glad to know that I could spend the night at his house anytime I wanted to. Usually we'd listen to U2, play Nintendo, and talk about which girls we thought were cute and which ones we thought were bitchy.

The topic of HIV never came up, even after Mark's mom told him the news. He was so laid-back about it—just like me—which is probably why we were so tight as friends. As cool as Mark was, there was one thing I couldn't forgive him for. "Hulk Hogan," he insisted, "is way better than Ric Flair."

Hogan personified a world in which the underdog never wins. Time after time he turned back challenges from his inferior foes, rubbing in their defeats with that post-match posedown. If Hogan was right, and the underdog didn't have a chance, that said to me that I was screwed in my own wrestling match with HIV.

In terms of "sick kids," my opinion of Hogan landed me distinctly in the minority. In the 1980s, he was the most-requested star for the Make-A-Wish Foundation—a group that tries to grant the final requests of kids with terminal illnesses—beating out Michael Jordan, Michael Jackson, and Michael Dukakis. I couldn't understand it. If life isn't fair, which is what kids with undesirable medical conditions often learn very early, doesn't it make more sense to idolize someone who *doesn't* play by the rules?

The essence of the Nature Boy's gritty spirit lurked much closer to my reality. Plus, he ended his matches covered in his own blood—definitely somebody a thinblood can relate to. He bent the rules to fit his own needs, and to survive HIV, I'd have to use the same guile that Ric Flair used in the ring to defeat my pet virus.

One day in eighth grade I overheard a couple of guys nearby talking.

"I know he's the one who has AIDS."

"It's gotta be him," the friend concurred.

When I turned around, eager to deny the accusation, I noticed they were not talking about me at all. Their attention was directed at a frail classmate who, to be honest, looked like every dying-of-AIDS character ever seen in the made-for-TV movies. Were I a devout Hulk Hogan fan, I would have come to his defense, saying, "Listen, brothers, he's not the one. *I'm* the student with HIV. See, not so easy to tell, is it? Well, don't be scared. Let's go sit down and talk about it."

Hulk Hogan encouraged his followers to obey his mantra, the Three Commandments of Hulkamania, which were: Say Your Prayers, Take Your Vitamins, and Listen to Your Parents. But in the cutthroat world of junior high school, you were a fool if you didn't follow the One Commandment of Adolescence: Every Zit-Faced, Pissed-Off Teenager for Himself.

"Yeah," I chimed in, desperate to deflect any AIDS-watching from myself. "You're probably right."

My dad loved professional wrestling, and like any good father he offered deeper thoughts than just what was happening on the programs. For instance, while watching the seven-foot-four, 500-pound Andre the Giant, the announc-

ers would say, "Andre the Giant can eat ten hamburgers in
one sitting . . . and that's just the appetizer!" Dad added his
own commentary: "Goddamm, I can't imagine what it looks
like after Andre takes a shit." When it came to HIV, Dad was
less inquisitive, because, like me, he didn't want to talk
about it. In fact, I can't remember ever talking with him
about AIDS when I was a kid.

Dad's fascination with the Giant's bowel movements
aside, I couldn't understand why Mom didn't join us when
wrestling was on. Maybe that's because her hero, Ryan
White, was a different personality type altogether.

Ryan White was born a thinblood, diagnosed with HIV,
and kicked out of school. His story, covered by the media
from day one, made Ryan a much-beloved hero for the
cause, because, by sharing his story, Ryan made AIDS a more
comfortable topic among legislators and rural communities.
He was changing the way Americans viewed the epidemic,
and my mom, along with millions of other people, fawned
over the cute, raspy-voiced kid from Indiana.

One morning, as I was polishing off a bowl of Lucky
Charms, Mom asked, "Do you want to do what Ryan White
does?"

When I thought about getting in on that action, I wondered how Ryan would react to my poor man's version of
himself. You never know how people are when the cameras
shut down, and if I treaded on his territory, I'd come face-

to-face with the original sooner or later. Probably backstage waiting to go on *The Phil Donahue Show.*

"Hey, hemo!"

I recognize the voice and turn around to see a shadowy figure approaching; it's Ryan White. And he doesn't look happy to see me. Menacingly, he begins to roll up the sleeves on his stone-washed blue-jean jacket. "Wait a minute," I say, my voice cracking with despair, "I can explain." Before I can finish, I'm on the ground, having been violently shoved to the hard concrete floor. Wiping the snot from my face, I look up to see Ryan standing above me. With one hand on his hip and the other combing his hair with what I initially feared to be a switchblade, Ryan speaks. "Don't you know? This is my turf." Lighting a cigarette, he takes a long, deliberate drag. That explains the rasp, I think. Grabbing me by the wrist, he extinguishes his cigarette on the palm of my hand, leaving a lifelong reminder that I messed with the wrong person. As I clutch my wounded paw to my chest, Ryan laughs and sneers through curled lips. "Now beat it, kid." With that he disappears through a curtain to an awaiting studio audience that erupts into a joyful standing ovation upon his arrival.

So maybe I was watching too much wrestling.

Granted, Ryan White wasn't the kind of guy to pummel a fellow thinblood into submission, but I wasn't the kind of kid who wanted to waste my breath on a bunch of morons who thought that HIV could be transmitted through handshakes or wedgies. So instead of putting it all out there—

taking my pet virus on the road—I opted for the stealthy route: more CIA than CNN.

At the time, I took Ryan's message a lot differently than the rest of the country. By being so public, the kid was kind of ratting me out, I thought, and I couldn't go to the bathroom in my own home without seeing him on the cover of *People*, smiling up at me, as if to say, "Hey, pal, how's the AIDS treatin' ya?" In my dream scenario, everyone, especially Ryan, would just shut up about the whole topic entirely, and that included my new HIV doctor.

Dr. Lyman Fisher was a short Canadian dude with white hair and a little Frenchie mustache. He'd zip around the hospital a mile a minute, and Mom, aware that he was one of the top hematologists in the country, would always remind me, "Dr. Fisher is a very important man."

But I didn't equate him with hemophilia; Dr. Lyman was my *HIV* doc. That's the real reason we went to see him, and the appointments weren't like the visits to Dr. Ron, who'd patch me up and send me home to collect a Slurpee and a toy on the ride back for my troubles. When I left Dr. Lyman, I was still just as HIV positive as I was when I got there, and I didn't understand the point of tracking my T cells if there wasn't anything they could do about them. So I argued with Mom all the way to Richmond, where Dr. Lyman worked at the Medical College of Virginia, cursing at her like a drunken sailor with Tourette's for the better part of the hour-long drive from Waynesboro, screaming words my dad would never *dream* of using in her presence. And that was pretty much the only time my mother and I spoke about HIV.

Once we got to Richmond, I'd small-talk with Dr. Lyman before he drew some blood, answering his questions with "yes" and "no" answers. Though I'd been stuck hundreds of times in my life, whenever blood was drawn in Richmond I got queasy and thought: This sample could be the one that shows that I'm about to take that dirt nap. Still, my mom rewarded me with a video game and a milkshake at Friendly's, and though those days started off rocky, they always ended quite well.

As time passed, I warmed up to Dr. Lyman, who would take my mom and me to the cafeteria across the street from MCV, a place called—no kidding—the Skull & Bones. I'd grab a wrestling magazine and eat my grilled-cheese sandwich as Mom and Dr. Lyman talked shop on AIDS research, statistics, and a bunch of other boring crap. Dr. Lyman scored big points when he'd say, "Eh, Shawn, go get another wrestling magazine, my treat."

Though I loathed my doctor's appointments and winced each time Ryan White came on TV, Mom felt the same trepidation with regard to Ric Flair and his on-air boasting. As I sat in front of the TV, my idol shouted: *"I can go all night long, baby! The ladies are lining up to take a ride on Space Mountain—wooooo!"*

Like any normal twelve-year-old, I wanted to follow in the footsteps of Ric Flair, not Ryan White. In my defense, it wasn't just the fictional persona of wrestling's dastardly darling that inspired me, but his own real-life battles as well.

In 1975, the same year I was born, Ric Flair was in a horrible plane crash that broke his back and killed another passenger. Just as his promising career started, he was suddenly laid up in a hospital bed, being told he would never wrestle again. Defying the medical prognosis, Flair rehabilitated himself and returned to the ring two years later: his hair bleached blond, his new physique adorned with expensive robes, and a cocky grin on his face that only comes from cheating death. In some bizarre way, Ric Flair allowed me to believe for the first time since my diagnosis that championship days lay ahead for me, too.

When Dad asked if I wanted to go see Ric Flair in nearby Richmond, I shouted, "Hell, yeah!" So I went with Kip and Dad to see the legend in action. Not only that, there was a chance that we might get to meet him in person!

Through his job with the state, Dad knew some of the security guards who worked the Richmond Coliseum, and by the combined powers of his gregarious personality and my own heart-wrenching ordeal, we were allowed to wait for the wrestlers in a private area as they entered the building. Nothing was promised, but I still couldn't believe my good fortune as a result of my bad fortune.

"Do you think Ric's coming?" I anxiously asked as we waited in the carport, getting pictures and autographs of many of the NWA's finest.

"Flair always wrestles in the last match," Dad said, "so he may arrive a little later than the others." Another car pulled up, but the Nature Boy didn't step out. "Just be patient, son."

As I paced around, I started to worry: Would Ric be as nice as the other wrestlers I'd met? Yeah, I kind of knew that the results were scripted, but the memory of John Stossell kept running through my head. During an interview, the star of 20/20's "Give Me a Break!" segment irritated a gruff wrestler by suggesting that the sport was fake, and he was repaid for his foolishness with a few brutal, open-handed palm strikes to the face. "Does that feel real?" the wrestler barked as Stossell likely rethought his career choice.

Seems that some of these guys have short fuses, and I wondered if Ric Flair would greet me by pounding the three of us into submission, or, worse still, ignoring me completely.

"It's him!"

The door of a Lincoln Town Car opened and out stepped the man. With a duffel bag slung over his shoulder and an empty cup of coffee in his hand, he looked more than ready for business. The four-time champion of the world approached and I grabbed my dad's arm as I stood trembling, a mere body slam away from greatness.

"Mr. Flair," my dad started. He referred to everyone as

"Mister," even a man who brutalized his adversaries with fists and chairs. "Could I get a picture of you with my son?"

Flair, who was already running late, stopped dead in his tracks and looked in our direction, his eyes obscured by sunglasses. A tinge of fear washed over me, and my life flashed before my eyes faster than a Ricky "The Dragon" Steamboat hip toss.

"Sure thing," Mr. Flair said disarmingly as he laid his bag, along with my anxiety, to rest at his feet. In my starstruck state I could only manage a few heartfelt words as my dad snapped a couple of pictures. "You're the best," I said. Ric Flair looked down and smiled, his infamous chest-chopping hand resting on my shoulder. "Thanks," he replied warmly.

As I stood there in amazement, the flash of Dad's camera went off and Flair was soon on his way to prepare for the evening's work. Once we took our seats, I put on my freshly purchased Ric Flair T-shirt and screamed as his forehead was busted open, leaving drops of his blood all around the ringside area. As we left, I wondered why the premises of the Richmond Coliseum, now baptized with the blood of Ric Flair, were not being roped off and declared sacred ground.

From that moment on I envisioned Ric Flair in a different light. How did he spend Christmas with his kids? Did the master of the figure-four leg-lock trade in his five-thousand-dollar robes for a Santa Claus hat and pass out presents while wearing a horrible sweater emblazoned with a reindeer,

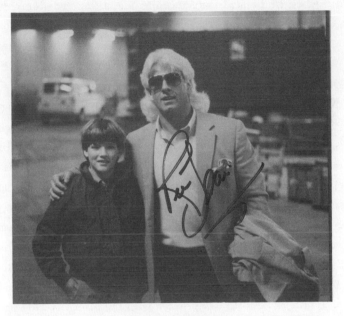

Surprisingly, no blood was shed when I met Ric Flair a few months after my HIV diagnosis.

complete with a blinking red nose? Did he grimace the same way he did when lifting his opponents up for a suplex as he did when he hoisted his son up to place the star atop the Christmas tree?

I don't really know how the Flairs spent their Christmas in 1987, when I was twelve. But I can tell you one thing: the Deckers should have had the shittiest Christmas this side of the Griswolds.

The rest of the year was strange. My pet virus was stressing out my family, and by the time Christmas rolled around, my dad had been out of the house for about two months, his eviction the result of a rocky patch for my parents that wasn't made any smoother by all the pressures that HIV placed on everyone: the doctor's visits with Mom, her decision to quit work for a few months, me staying home from school, and the fact that I might not be around much longer. In short, things sucked.

Dad became mildly depressed with the thought of losing me, and even though she shared his concern, Mom thought, "Oh, Bud will get over this soon." But as the months passed, her patience with him dwindled, and one night she said maybe he should move out. Dad shocked us all when he actually did.

Dad's nearby apartment was small and obviously meant to be temporary. There was also a flagrant display there of one of Dad's greatest passions, junk food: the refrigerator was stacked with ice cream sandwiches, and the cabinets overflowed with chips, candy bars, and various delectable treats. "Help yourself, son." I'd dig in, stopping only when I felt ill. When I'd leave, Dad would say, "Tell your mother I love her."

Mom explained the whole situation. "Right now your father and I need a break," she said, though she was mum when I asked if they'd ever get back together. "Would you rather us be happy apart or miserable together?"

That Christmas, the family spent the holiday together, and the misery factor, for me at least, seemed to be at a minimum. In fact, Kip and I were rolling in gifts, because not only did Mom load us down that year, but Dad also arrived with a car-full of gifts. Mountains of presents surrounded us, and my mom just glared at Dad as he made another trip outside to the car, returning with another bag of presents. "He just wants to beat me," she stewed.

Our Christmas Gift Olympics—where the goal was to receive the most gifts—had originated at my grandparents' house, where all the aunts and uncles on my mother's side— four sets, to be exact—would gather with their offspring. There was no drawing of names; you could buy for whomever you wanted, and some people got more than others. The gift opening proceeded from youngest to oldest and continued until the last gift was opened. By the end of December 25, you knew where you stood.

Every year it came down to Grandmother versus Grandad in a gift-getting fight to the finish. Grandmother was like the

Hulk Hogan of this competition, and every year, at around the three-hour mark, it ended the same way: with Grandad going down in defeat, having to settle for the silver medal.

But not in '87. When the top contender reached under his chair for that one last present that wasn't there, someone made an unusual declaration. "Grandad, you're out! It's Shawn's turn!" Everybody had the same idea that Christmas: double-up on the "sick kid," as it may be his last appearance at the Christmas Olympics. No one suspected that the upstart rookie with no future could go all the way.

The family was on the edge of their seats, couches, and various spots on the floor in varying degrees of comfort. Package-for-package, I was hanging with the tough old bird, and the momentum shifted at a feverish pace. "I see your quilt and raise you a Nintendo game!" I had a real chance to bring new, tainted blood to the throne of Family Matriarch.

But soon I found out what Grandad discovered years before I was born, and with my last gift behind me, she coasted to a narrow two-gift win. "Put that in your pipe and smoke it, sonny," she yelled, balling up the last of the wrapping paper and pelting me in the head with it.

That Christmas I relished the attention and all of the presents that were given to me, and I was starting to come to terms with my pet virus, slowly emerging from my self-imposed exile from school. At the end of the year, I had two New Year's resolutions: find a girlfriend and make it to the next holiday season.

the silent treatment

A few months into the new year my parents got back together. It was around the same time I was starting to become social again. They let me throw little parties of the soda, movies, and board game variety that were well attended. One night we broke out the classic game of spin the bottle, and if any of the girls who were present knew I was HIV positive, none showed any concern or refused to give me a little peck when the bottle commanded they do so.

Though I was getting back into the social scene, the trend of setting my own slack school schedule continued, and through the rest of seventh grade I continued to rack up record "sick days." Teachers—all of whom were informed of my HIV status for safety reasons, should I bleed—must have

sympathized with my situation, because I passed each semester. With everyone distracted by HIV, another condition
stealthily began to take over my life: RDS (restless dick
syndrome).

All the signs were there: mid-class erections, wet dreams,
and masturbation. I was doing as well as could be expected
with my pet virus, but the RDS had quickly developed into
full-blown puberty, and I forgot all about the fear of developing the AIDS blotches of KS when I noticed a zit on my chin
and a patch of hair under my arms.

Though I was starting to think about AIDS less, I was beginning to wonder about French kissing: Could I partake
without killing anyone? I was too embarrassed to ask my
parents, so I asked Dr. Lyman. "Well, Shawn," he started,
surprised that I'd initiated a conversation about HIV. "If you
French-kiss someone and your gums are bleeding, and they
have an open sore in their mouth . . . then, yes, there is a
small chance that the virus can be transmitted."

Good enough for me!

He also added that, as of yet, there'd been no reported
cases of HIV being transmitted this way. Which made me
wonder: Who *would* really kiss someone if they were bleeding from the mouth?

Later, as I watched Ric Flair strutting down the aisle
toward the ring with six women—three on each arm—my gaze
drifted from the TV and I imagined, for the first time, that

someday I, too, could be at the helm of such a bevy of beauties. Heck, I'd settle for one.

Eighth grade started out much better than seventh had, and I accomplished a goal that no other Decker male has come close to besting: four girlfriends in one school year, two of whom I French-kissed! Kelly was first.

Our little case of puppy love was great. Kelly came over to my house for Ping-Pong matches, and I went with her to cheerleading practice. We even went public with our romance, attending the 1950s-themed dance together, her in a poodle skirt and me sporting the greaser look, my hair slicked back and one of Mom's empty cigarette packs rolled up in the sleeve of my white T-shirt.

One day she was over at my house, and as her mother honked the horn to pick her up, Kelly decided that it was time to give her boyfriend a little pick-me-up. I couldn't have been more shocked when, as we were saying goodbye, with her mom waiting in the driveway, Kelly grabbed me and stuck her tongue in my mouth. Well, on second thought, I *could* be more shocked. Like the time she asked me the most dreaded question imaginable.

"Do you have AIDS?"

We were at school, in between classes, and Kelly was crying. Someone had told her about me; she being a grade younger, the information took a while to reach her through her classmates.

I blankly stared at my Chuck Taylors, mute as we stood in the middle of the hallway. The Love Boat that I'd been effortlessly navigating up to this point had clipped a massive chunk of ice and my head sunk deep into my chest. Fortunately, a friend of mine overheard the drama and threw me a flotation device.

"No," the voice said, sternly. It was Denial!

Like other teenagers, I kept certain friends for certain situations: my video-game buddies for hours of mindless enjoyment, my mall rats for social interaction, my sleepover pals for the weekends, and Denial to help me out with HIV. Growing up, I'd never seen a more effective solution to a nagging problem than "the silent treatment," and I couldn't think of a better way to deal with a life-threatening, incurable illness.

One of the unfortunate side effects of my silent-treatment plan was that when I started dating, others would meddle with my hear-no-virus, see-no-virus, speak-no-virus tactic.

After Denial stepped in and told Kelly no, my gaze lifted from my shoes to my girlfriend, and much to my relief, her face now bore the expression of a lottery winner. "Thank God," she sighed, firmly squeezing my hand before rushing off to beat the bell for her next class.

Moments later, as I plopped down in my desk, I wondered . . . *If I told her the truth, would things change? Would she dump me? Would I no longer be the recipient of those sweet kisses?*

As I struggled for an answer, Denial put his arm around me and said, "Wait a minute, jackrabbit, you didn't lie."

While I was humbled by his concern for me, we were obviously less than forthcoming with the information at hand. Undeterred, Denial asked:

"You're HIV positive, right?"

"Yeah," I said in a hushed tone, wondering where this ridiculous question was headed.

"Well," he continued, "she asked if you had AIDS. HIV is *the virus that causes AIDS.* Remember? Technically speaking, we told the truth."

Kelly and I were visiting her grandparents in the country-side—acres of cows and corn along miles of one-lane road—safely removed from the hallways of junior high. When we got there, I noticed a wolflike creature chained down in the barn, gnawing on a piece of red meat. The family "dog," as they called it, must have had a taste for thinblood, because when he saw me he gave chase. I ran for my life, and that chain did its job, snapping the beast back.

"Are you okay?" Kelly asked frantically. I thought I was. Then I looked down at my sock. It was drenched in blood, and a thin stream led up to the back of my knee, where I'd been nipped.

I wasn't that comfortable at the sight of blood streaming from anywhere besides my nose, and the fact that we were out in Heehaw-land, miles away from factor VIII and the vile syrup Amicar, made me nervous. Kelly's family took me inside and bandaged me up, putting pressure on my leg. I didn't even think much about HIV, and soon I was back home.

Turns out that while I was bleeding, Kelly's mom called my parents, and my dad ratted on me by disclosing my HIV status.

"You did what?"

Of course, Dad had no choice. I was bleeding all over the place and it was the right thing to do, but I was pissed. This was my secret, my silent-treatment plan, and it was working. I could deal with little bastards running around the hallway telling secrets that no one could prove. But my dad?

Turned out that Kelly didn't care; she stayed with me. Her mom didn't flip out, either, and even wrote a nice note to my mother, informing her that I was being prayed for and was welcome in their house anytime. Meanwhile, her grandparents were worried about whether I'd infected their beloved bloodthirsty dog with AIDS. I didn't. Even if I had, I wouldn't have lost any sleep over that one.

But the relationship with Kelly wasn't the same anymore. When we kissed I no longer felt like a boyfriend; I felt like a charity case. I wasn't about to pour my heart out over HIV—I wouldn't have known what to say about it, anyway, and it killed me that she knew. Every time I saw Kelly, I thought about AIDS, so there was only one solution: I broke up with her.

"See what happened?" Denial asked. "Can't say I didn't warn ya."

After Kelly, I held back a little more with my other girlfriends, one of whom broke up with me because I *wouldn't* kiss her. I guess you could say that the next great love of my life wasn't a girl; it was music.

Upon entering high school, Mark and I formed a band, The Demonic Doves. We started it after an unsuccessful episode with the indoor track team that we cut short with a jog to Hardees. "Fuck that," Mark said as we shared an order of fries. "What's 'indoor' about running laps in the rain?" So maybe we weren't cut out for relay races, but having just gotten our musical instruments—he a drum kit and me a Casio keyboard—Mark and I were ready for the cover of *Rolling Stone*.

The fact that The Demonic Doves couldn't make it through a song and had no lead singer didn't matter; blind ambition would be our bread and butter. Armed with a bass player and our friend Ryan on guitar, we came up with a mash-up single, combining each band member's favorite song: "New Year's Day" by U2, "Sunshine of Your Love" by Cream, "Strangelove" by Depeche Mode, and a few bars of Jimi Hendrix thrown in for seasoning.

During a cassette-tape recording session, tragedy almost struck the Doves. There was a thunderstorm raging outside and Ryan was electrocuted through his electric guitar when lightning struck nearby. The sound of his bloodcurdling screams was caught on tape, and we delightedly listened to it over and over again. Ryan Almarode survived this high-voltage jam session with The Demonic Doves unscathed, but around the same time, Mom's hero, Ryan White, passed away.

Mom told me the sad news, her face washed out and her cheeks sunken; this was a big shock to her, but not so much to me. Ryan White always looked thin and frail. And every time I saw an article on him it said things like "Young Boy Dying from AIDS," or something to that effect. What was shocking was that, in her grief over Ryan, Mom contacted the Make-A-Wish Foundation. When she told me, I was confused.

"Don't I have to, like, be dying soon to get a wish?" I asked, confused yet enticed by the offer.

"Well," Mom explained, "with HIV nobody knows what will happen. Why not do something fun while you're still healthy and can enjoy it?"

Mom was feeding me a line to make it happen. She was convinced that I wouldn't live to see Christmas that year. Not because I was getting sick, but because Ryan White died. If God could take Ryan, then none of the rest of us thinbloods stood much of a chance.

Since I was fourteen at the time, you can guess what I *really* wanted, but I was savvy enough to deduce that the Make-A-Wish Foundation wouldn't set a kid up with a Brigitte Nielsen booty call. So I asked for the next best thing: to meet Depeche Mode, my favorite band. If I'd thought it through a little more, I might have chosen Mötley Crüe—they would *definitely* have gotten me laid.

Fate smiled upon my wish: Depeche Mode was on tour for their 1990 album, *Violator*, and would soon be in Virginia. The band accepted the request, and I was allowed to bring Mark. This wasn't just an opportunity to meet the Beatles of electronic music, it was a chance to break out the Beatles of Waynesboro, The Demonic Doves, into the mainstream by slipping Depeche Mode a demo tape.

Before the concert, Mark and I were whisked backstage to meet the band. We walked into a room, and each member of Depeche Mode politely introduced himself. (As if I didn't know who they were!) This was a couple of years before the lead singer, Dave Gahan, began his descent into heroin addiction, and on the day of my Wish he was on his best behavior. He would have been cool even on smack. I was too nervous to finish a potato chip, which I wrapped in a napkin and set by the hors d'oeuvres table, hoping Depeche Mode didn't notice. I was blowing my Wish, but Mark was on top of his game, asking keyboardist Alan Wilder what it was like to perform live for millions of people before slyly slipping him the Demonic demo tape, which must have gotten lost, since we never heard back from the band or their record label.

While I was meeting my favorite band, Kip, sixteen, was reporting for his first day of duty as an employee of McDonald's. He stopped by my room that morning for a photo opportunity, proudly standing beside me in his uniform, but I

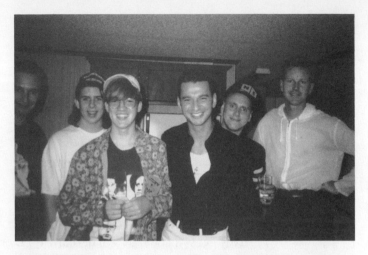

Catching up with Depeche Mode with my best friend, Mark.

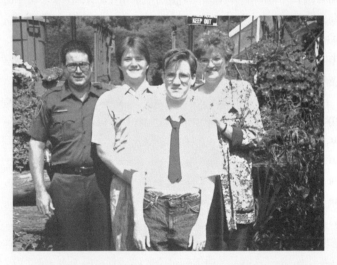

The Deckers in 1989, not as creepy as we appear.

was too lazy and disinterested to get out of my waterbed. I rolled over, shook his hand, and smiled for the camera, then went back to sleep. "Shawn," my mom said as they were exiting, "just wait until *your* first day of work!"

Throughout high school my job wasn't to prepare Happy Meals, it was defending Depeche Mode's sexual orientation. "Did you know that 'Depeche Mode' is French for 'We're fags'?" said Steven, an obnoxious upperclassman who targeted me for insults because I proudly wore Depeche Mode T-shirts to school. Not about to let some jerk make fun of the Mode, I shot back, "They're not gay, dumbass—they're European."

There weren't many "out" people at Waynesboro High School. One of my classmates, it was assumed, had to be gay. He was a standout in chorus and exhibited all the feminine mannerisms one equates, rightly or wrongly, with homosexuality. One day in class he got in an argument with a jock, who said, "Shut up, you faggot!" And the teacher didn't say a word.

So if Depeche Mode were straight, why didn't they have any facial hair? Or a drummer? On top of those oddities, they wore lots of leather and didn't use distorted electric guitars, either. Plus, Martin Gore would occasionally take the stage in makeup and a skirt, but he didn't write killer metal tunes like Judas Priest.

Maybe I was wrong.

But I didn't care. Depeche Mode inspired me to conquer

the world of music, and if they enjoyed the intimate company of other men, who was I to judge?

Pretty soon I tired of defending the private lives of Depeche Mode altogether. "So what if they are," I said to Steven, who befriended me when he discovered that I was a Ric Flair fan.

Years later I learned the truth: Depeche Mode *weren't* gay. They were a bunch of skirt-chasin' straight dudes. I was stunned. Still, I found it in my heart to forgive them for enjoying the intimate company of women, something I wouldn't experience until the tenth grade.

Every day before fourth period I saw her and wondered if she noticed me, as well. Unable to work up the nerve to approach her, I safely admired from a distance. After two months of what could be considered stalking, I made my move. Though I was extremely nervous about how the infiltration would be received, I dropped my handwritten letter of admiration into her locker. It read something like this:

Hey Jennifer,

My name is Shawn. I'm friends with Benjy; he has science class with you. Please don't judge my character by the antics of those I choose to hang around with . . . just kidding, Benjy is a great guy. Anyway, this is rambling, I just

wanted to see if you'd like to chat sometime? If so, feel free
to give me a call or write back.

Later, Shawn

For the rest of the afternoon I sweated profusely. Had she
ever noticed me during all the buildup, or had I only imagined some kind of connection? At times, I could have sworn
that she was timing her water-fountain visits in order to get
a better look at me as I entered my adjoining class. After a
longer than usual day I opened my locker and a piece of
paper tumbled out—a response! Frantically I unfolded the
note, grasping it tightly in my clammy hands:

If you want to talk, give me a call this weekend.

Bye, Jen

Bingo!

I called Jen and we spoke for close to three hours without
a second of awkward silence. Turns out that she had been admiring me from afar after all. Best of all, her favorite band
was Depeche Mode, too! When Jen saw the picture of me
with the Mode in my locker, her jaw hit the floor. "Holy shit,
Shawn! How did you meet them?" Not wanting my dream
girl to know that I was on the Make-A-Wish Death List, I
said, "Oh, my dad knew one of the security guards."

Jen was a stellar student, and as we began to date, some of

that began to rub off on me. "You can get an A in English, Shawn," she said. "That should be your best subject!" After some tutoring—which mainly consisted of her cutting our phone calls short during the week so I could study—I went from a C to an A-minus. "See!" she said enthusiastically.

While Jen had my best academic interests at heart, Mr. Prick, one of my teachers, attempted to give me an education of an entirely different kind.

Prick, like all of my other teachers, knew about my pet virus, and he was infamous for his snide and inappropriate remarks. "Man, I was at the basketball game the other night, and Megan was sitting in front of me . . . I could hardly concentrate on the game with those legs staring up at me!" Indeed, the legs in question were a startling pair, but they belonged to an eleventh-grade student. Still, the worst offense came at my expense: a ten-minute speech detailing the slow and agonizing death of the AIDS patient. "A lot of people think it's fast," Mr. Prick said, shaking his head. "It most certainly is not."

I wasn't sure what this had to do with the course he was teaching, but I knew it was a direct attack meant specifically for me. Speaking up or leaving the room would have effectively announced my HIV status, so I just sat there, trying to ignore Mr. Prick. Though I have to admit, thinking about Megan's legs helped.

Good study habits weren't the only thing I learned from

Jen, and soon I spent every weekday in anticipation of the weekends, when we'd either go to a movie, grab a bite to eat somewhere, or end up hanging out at my house watching TV in my room, which is where Jen made her move.

"Is this all right?" she asked as her hand made a move southward. "Uh, sure," I said. Before I knew it, things were hotter and heavier than I was prepared for. Touching led to kissing, which led to more kissing, which led to oral sex.

I didn't really know what the risks were, though I'd heard that oral sex wasn't nearly as dangerous as intercourse. Since I had no condoms on hand, my solution was simple: just don't come. And it worked. When Jen left after some fooling around, I just finished things off in the bathroom.

Since my guy friends weren't hanging around so much, my mom got suspicious.

"Shawn, are you having sex?" she asked.

Eight years before President Clinton's fling with Monica was revealed, I was being grilled about the same thing, and, like Bill, I denied the charge when backed into a corner. Mom followed up with another probing question. "Have you spoken to her about hemophilia and HIV?"

"Not yet," I answered. "But I will."

Was I putting Jen at risk? The last thing I would want to do is infect someone else with HIV, but if there weren't any bodily fluids involved, how could it be so dangerous? As hard as it was, I called the National AIDS Hotline to ask a stranger about oral sex. "Oral sex is not safe!" he told me. "Uh . . . is it safer than intercourse?" "No! It's not safe!" I wasn't getting anywhere, but I'd heard that, statistically, oral sex was safer than intercourse. There was one more nugget of info I needed. "Well, what if you don't come?" The guy lost his patience. *"It's not safe! Ever!"*

I'm not sure what I expected to hear, but I felt like if I'd suggested cutting off my penis altogether, he wouldn't have talked me away from the scissors.

At my next doctor's appointment, the usual banter involved a new subject. "Eh, I hear you're seeing a girl." Great. Now Dr. Lyman was in on the interrogation of my personal life, but I still didn't admit to having sex. I knew that Jen needed to know about my pet virus, that she deserved that much. But disclosing wasn't as easy as everyone was making it out to be. "Let me know if you need my help," Dr. Lyman said. Oh, sure, maybe a double date with my doctor and his wife that ends with a big surprise: Hey, Jen, your boyfriend has HIV!

In a perfect world, I would have told Jen before the relationship got physical. But things moved along so quickly—too quickly for rational thinking, I rationalized. In my mind, everyone knew about my HIV status anyway, and even though most of my closest friends did, it never came up—not with Mark, or anyone else. Which meant that, until Jen, my plot to expunge my pet virus from my life by not speaking about it had worked, even in a place like Waynesboro, where word travels fast. But, of course, I found a girl who didn't know, which I thought would make things easier. Boy, was I wrong.

On Friday I'll tell her. After we go out, I'll have a talk with her in the car when she drops me off at home.

The plan sounded great on Tuesday, but as the weekend closed in, my resolve weakened, and I couldn't end a perfectly charming evening with, "I had a great time . . . By the way, I have HIV. Goodnight!"

Since I didn't talk to anyone about the dating drama, only one of my friends, Denial, knew about my torment, and he showed up to offer some much-needed advice. "Hey, you're not doing anything too risky," he said. "And don't let everyone get in your business. They're just jealous because you're young and in love. You're happy, man! So what's the big problem here?"

Mom sensed I wasn't going to hold up my end of the bargain and warned, "If you don't tell Jen yourself, then I will."

The best chance to tell Jen came on a weekend when her parents were going out of town. This provided the ideal scenario; we'd be alone for two whole days. Like any good friend, Mark hooked me up with an alibi for the evening—as well as a condom. But as it turned out, I'd need only the former. My intentions were honorable, but I soon decided that Jen's vision of how events would unfold was much more enticing than mine: she wanted to have intercourse.

As we were lying in bed after a night of playing cards, watching movies, and drinking loads of cherry-flavored soda, things started to heat up. I put on the condom, but each time my penis got anywhere near Jen I cooled down: my conscience was cock-blocking me.

I really felt horrible, and Denial was nowhere to be found. When Jen asked what was wrong, I gave her an honest answer. "I'm not ready." "Do you love me?" "Yes," I answered, fully aware that my reluctance had more to do with caring about her than not. A few weeks later, when I was in my bedroom—alone—my dad peeked his head in.

"Shawn, get your coat."

"What's going on?" I asked.

"We're going to Jennifer's house."

Dad explained that Mom was already there, and that she'd told Jen's family about my pet virus. Mom knew I'd never be able to, and Dr. Lyman worried that if Jen and I were having sex, as they'd suspected, there was a risk of transmitting the virus. Betrayed, I unhooked my seat belt and hoped some kind angel would slam into the passenger side of the car with a tank, because I realized that my relationship with Jen—my first true love—was over.

Upon arrival, Dad went inside to join the other parents, and Jen and I took a slow walk around the block, stopping to sit on the steps of a church. "They know *everything*," she said, having just lived through the worst hour of her life. We were both in a state of shock, sitting side by side as our parents discussed our fate. I'd never felt so helpless.

Not only had her parents discovered that their daughter

was having sex, but now they knew her boyfriend was a posi-toid. Oh, and one more thing, *he didn't tell her.* I felt so bad for Jen, she had to get tested for HIV (the test came back negative) and vaccinated for hepatitis B, and even after all of that, I still didn't talk to her about HIV.

After we weren't allowed to see each other anymore, Jen and I sneaked around for a few weeks, but she wasn't enjoying my silence about all the things I should have been saying. So, in a poetic twist, I wasn't even told that I was dumped; it was assumed that I knew.

"You guys ruined my social life," I told my parents, angry with them for causing my downfall. "I am human and I need to be loved!" My outlook suffered not only as a result of having been dumped by my first love; I was also OD-ing on the Smiths.

The summer picked up when I got a visit from my old bandmate from The Demonic Doves, Ryan Almarode. Like Mark, he knew I was a positoid, but we never talked about it. While I was dating Jen, he became the leader of a group of harmless goons who were dubbed "The Almarodies." He heard through the grapevine that I was once again a bache-lor, and when I opened the front door, Ryan said, "Man, I'm really sorry you got dumped." Then his face lit up with a big smile, and he added, "But I'm so happy for me! I thought my summer was going to suck!"

It wasn't as fun as making out with Jen, but hanging out with the lanky Ryan—who was just as selfish as me—was the next-best thing. He habitually raided his parents' liquor cabinet, and the partying was fun, until the morning when, after a bender, I woke up and Ryan—whom I'd been sharing a bottle of vodka with in a dugout—was nowhere to be found. Then I noticed that I wasn't in Ryan's room, where I'd planned on spending the night.

I was in the hospital.

"You were in a coma!" Mom said, fucking with me.

"I was just sleeping, Mom."

The truth, which was somewhere in between, was that I blacked out after being found by the police around one a.m., puking my guts out and babbling incoherently outside of a church. I was taken to the hospital, and Ryan was taken to jail to sleep it off. My preferential treatment was the result of one of the officers recognizing me and calling my dad in to assess the situation. "You looked like a damn animal," Dad said.

With his job as a beer cop, Dad had been humiliated professionally, so maybe I got him back for his part in ruining my social life, after all.

Even though my decision-making skills weren't exactly peaking, my parents were cool enough to know that Ryan and I made a mistake, and they continued to let us hang out together. In fact, when he had trouble at home a few months later, they let him move in with us for close to eight weeks. Still, after my drunken escapade, it took a couple of weeks— and a strange twist of fate—to get back on the good side of my father.

As Ryan and I were walking the half-mile from my house to his, a car drove by and one of the passengers yelled at us. Thinking it was one of Ryan's Almarodies, I hollered back.

"Oh shit," Ryan said. He recognized the car, which pulled around the corner and stopped right beside us. It was a group of four black guys, and they wanted to beat up some white kids. They'd already racked up two by the time they came upon us.

Two guys jumped out of the car, and I knew the person who squared up in front of me. "Sorry about that, Tyrell," I explained. "I thought you were one of my friends."

Tyrell and I had had problems in school before. He was always trying to bully white kids, and a small group that he ran with were obsessed with Compton and "the man." I thought it was kind of funny, though I wisely kept my laughs to myself. "You're racist," Tyrell would say in class, mean-muggin' for no reason. I almost got the sense that he was hoping everyone *was* a racist, so he'd have something to fight about.

But my peace-making efforts met a deaf ear. "You don't know who we are," Tyrell said. By this time, his cohort was already pounding Ryan, who was doing his best to roll with the punches and provide a bad target. Not me; I planted my feet and accepted my fate.

"Sure I do," I said. "You're Tyrell. We had art class together last year."

"No," he corrected, acting even more gangsta than necessary. *"You don't . . ."*

Of course, I knew what he was getting at. *Don't tell anyone what's about to happen.* He must have seen this in a movie somewhere, but I saw what was happening to Ryan, and I figured I wasn't going to play by the script. "Yes, I do, Tyrell. We also had science together two years ago."

By now he was getting frustrated, and I kept talking because it was better than being a punching bag. Plus, I was intent on making this the most awkward, emasculating beatdown he'd ever issue. "You're also friends with Tyrone . . . Hey, what's he up to tonight?"

Done with the small talk, Tyrell struck me in the eye and then on the side of the head. I love boxing, and to his credit, it was a pretty snappy one-two. Ryan's guy was done and back in the car, and my buddy seemed to be okay. The rest of the squad were getting antsy waiting for Tyrell, who hopped in for the quick getaway. I should have implemented my silent-treatment plan, but I wasn't done talking. As if we'd just enjoyed cookies and milk at Sunday school, I shouted to the car. "See you at school on Monday . . . *Tyrell.*"

"What did you say?" he yelled back.

"Oh," I said, bracing myself for one more shot as he got out of the car and menacingly walked toward me. "I thought you were done already."

With that, Tyrell landed an open-handed slap to the ear, busting my eardrum. The car was already moving, so he ran to it, jumped in, and disappeared into the night. My ear, ringing worse than it might after a Demonic Doves band practice, was buzzing, and I had to turn my head sideways to hear Ryan, who wasn't hurt as bad. "Man," he said, "what the fuck were you doing?" By now we were both laughing as the blood dried on our faces. "You know what, Shawn?" Ryan said, turning kind of thoughtful. "I've always *wondered* what it would be like to get my ass kicked."

My family wasn't so amused.

When I showed up at home, my eye swollen and globs of blood in my ear, pandemonium broke lose. Kip, eighteen, had been one of the bigger guys on the high school football team, plus he sported a nasty-looking mullet. In his eyes, this was attempted murder, and before anyone knew it, he'd scrambled through the house, found a gun, and charged out the door, as his girlfriend—and future wife, Deanna—screamed like a banshee and gave chase.

Fortunately, Kip didn't get very far that night.

But my mom—sans gunplay—was ready to battle. Especially when she found out that a tire on my car had been slashed at school. Noticing a group of my classmates in the school parking lot, Mom walked over to them and said, "I've got a hundred dollars for the first person who tells me who did this." And the following week Ryan and I testified in juvenile court about the altercation.

Both my mom and the court must have had a calming effect on Tyrell's demeanor. From then on, he opened doors for me at school and said hi in the hallway. I assumed it was because of the stand we made in court, or perhaps he respected my machismo that night when everything went down. I later found out the truth. After the incident, one of my relatives pulled up to a group of black teenagers in a grocery-store parking lot, hopped out of his truck, and said: "You tell Tyrell that if he ever messes with Shawn Decker again, he's going to be one dead nigger!"

The downside of getting bloodied at the fists of Tyrell was getting bloodied at the fists of Tyrell, which showed me that racism cuts both ways in Waynesboro. The upside of getting bloodied at the fists of Tyrell was that, in my father's eyes, I was once again a sympathetic character, and no longer the drunken miscreant with the rolled-back eyes throwing up outside a church; this was well worth a few hard-earned wallops to the head.

my so-called
midlife crisis

Getting dumped, trashed beyond belief, and beaten up was cathartic, and by summer's end I was ready to turn over a new leaf, which meant I had to distance myself from friends who were still partying hard. When the new school year rolled around, Kip was off to college, which meant that all parental eyes were on me. And in the previous three months I'd pretty much punched out all the tabs on my fuck-up card.

During the first week of eleventh grade, Mr. Taylor, a Vietnam vet with a dry sense of humor, instructed our English class to write an essay. "I'd like to know a little bit about who you are, so write whatever you like." This assignment was the closest I ever came to disclosing my HIV status in high school, and though I avoided writing about my pet virus specifically, I danced around it vaguely. Since all the teachers and staff were informed of my status, it was easy for Mr. Taylor to read between the lines. In my essay, I also made an admiring reference to the stunning exchange student from Denmark, Maja.

The day after I turned in my essay, Mr. Taylor passed out a seating chart. Most of the students were irritated at having to gather their belongings and move to a new seat, but not me; I was right beside the girl from Denmark. The teacher shot me a knowing smile, and his helpful hookup worked; Maja and I became friends, and that fall we went to the homecoming dance. But I was still shell-shocked from the Jen experience and didn't really pursue anyone that year. To be honest, I didn't want the trouble. Plus, I knew that I needed to talk about my pet virus if I ever wanted to get serious with someone. I came close a couple of times, but still couldn't say that I had HIV.

My senior year I was crowned Homecoming King. For six years my HIV status floated through the hallways, never confirmed by me, and this may have been a way for my classmates to say that they—unlike some adults over the years— were cool with it, and instead of crowning a sweaty football player, they made the wiseass, Depeche Mode–loving positoid king.

On homecoming night, all my friends rushed the field to pick me up and carry me around for a victory lap as my family cheered from the stands. I tried to parlay the fame into a bid for class president, but was undermined when a few teachers started telling my classmates that the president is in charge of planning the ten-year high school reunion, the implication being that a vote for me would be wasted. So, in contrast to my landslide Homecoming King victory, where I was the beneficiary of lowered expectations for my longevity, in this election those same expectations worked against me.

I recovered from my first and last foray into politics just in time for graduation, though I can't say I was as fired up for this one as I was for my elementary school ceremony. As king, I voiced my objections to Mom, thinking she'd understand how lame it was and let me skip out. "Now, Shawn," she said, giving me a glimpse of the eye of the tiger that had defeated the evil forces of the Waynesboro school system six years earlier, "I don't ask you to do much. But you *will* be going to school on that day."

So I put on the purple cap and gown, and looked just like all the rest of my classmates, who were celebrating a stepping-stone toward the future. I wasn't like them, though. What does a positoid do after high school? Of course, my family was just as happy as everyone else, if not happier, because I wasn't supposed to be alive to graduate. I hadn't really studied since the sixth grade, so I knew college was out, but if I wanted a taste of the campus life, I'd just visit my brother at Ferrum College, a couple of hours away. The only time I second-guessed my decision not to seek higher education was when,

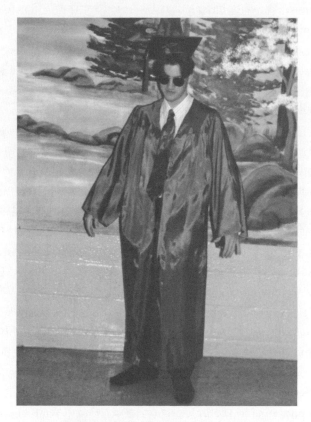

**High school graduation day, 1993—
officially too cool for school.**

after a few beers at one of Kip's parties, I disclosed my status for the first time to one of my brother's female college pals. "I know," she said, having heard it from Kip. Then we made out and she let me feel her up.

Aside from that enlightening and encouraging experience, one of the things that kept me sane the summer after high school was the fact that my new best friend, Josh, still had two years of high school left.

Meeting Josh, in many ways, was a lifesaver; he shared my sense of humor, and Waynesboro had yet to erode his soul. I joined Josh's social circle of sophomores, renting kung fu movies, playing video games all night, and just goofing off. I was sure they had heard the rumors that I was a positoid, but no one ever called me out on it. Josh's mom taught at the high school, so she definitely knew, but she didn't care that by the end of the year I was practically living at their house, an unofficial member of the family. And with two more years of high school to go for Josh, I kicked my feet back, relieved that I didn't have to worry about what to do next—socially, professionally, or otherwise.

It wasn't that I *never* had a plan. I did. It's just that the music career never took off the way I'd anticipated. I was supposed to be set for life by my twenties, but at age eighteen another health crisis hampered my career trajectory and further lessened my odds of living to see that Grammy nomination.

Home alone, I was fiddling around on my synthesizers,

surrounded by Depeche Mode posters. I'd started to get pretty good, but on this night, instead of feeling a groove, I felt a nosebleed coming on. A slow one drips at the tempo of, say, a ballad. As I leaned over the toilet, the pace was more reminiscent of speed metal. *Drip-drip-drip-drip.*

I dialed up Dr. Ron, who met me at the emergency room.

It was good to see my old friend again. He did his best to stop the bleed, but silver nitrate sticks weren't doing the trick. Mom and Dad, who came home to a note I scribbled to inform them that I was at the hospital, arrived with my aunt Amy, who brought some factor VIII from home because her son—my cousin—is also a thinblood.

After factoring up, I picked up where I left off with my music, but the tune was about to change.

Dr. Lyman had been testing me for a couple of years, and was amazed because most of his positoid patients were co-infected with hepatitis C, a virus that affects the liver. This latest viral infection craze was sweeping the bleeding-disorder community, and until that trip to the hospital, I'd been lucky. But I finally joined the club when I received that treatment from a product whose label read: "Warnings: NONE."

The hep C diagnosis hit me harder than HIV. When you're a kid, you just figure that your parents can deal with anything and somehow fix it. Now, as an adult, I was much more aware of the potential for disaster, and I thought about my liver rotting inside my body to the point where my side started to hurt. Great, I thought, poking around and trying to remember which side my liver was actually on. I survive HIV, and then a *nosebleed* ends up killing me.

The next morning I woke up feeling great and, to my own surprise, I rationalized the situation: If my pet virus couldn't finish me off, then why should I worry about this new guy?

Despite my sunny attitude, I was more tired than usual, a symptom of hepatitis C infection as well as of the progression of HIV. My parents noticed, and one night at dinner Mom and Dad started talking about Social Security Disability. This came as a surprise to me, for, in my mind, I could climb Mount Everest if I had to. But as I listened, I knew they were right. I wasn't realistic about my limitations, or the fact that when I used to stay home from school, some of those days I really *wasn't* feeling up to it. And, honestly, who would hire someone who left early every other day and took ten days of work off a month?

After high school, Mom and Dad gave me money all the time, so that wasn't an issue. But if I qualified for disability, I'd have my own money, and my parents—who were already putting Kip and his girlfriend, Deanna, through college—wouldn't have to support me on top of that. It seemed stupid not to swallow my pride and do it, so I put in my application, which was approved.

The first check for $400 came, and I felt really uncomfortable as I drove to the bank. At the drive-thru window my palms were sweaty and my eyes shifty. When the teller asked me how she could help me, I couldn't make eye contact. Just placed the check in the tube and said, "Cash this." I may as well have had a pistol in my hand and pantyhose on my head.

The cash seemed cold and hard, but so was the truth: after years of pretending, I wasn't so normal after all. None of my friends were on disability; and even though the check itself read "Disability," I still didn't consider myself "disabled." An easier word to handle would have been "unabled." Through a combination of my lack of studying, the bleeding disorder, my miserable work ethic, and pitiful energy levels, I was *unable* to be a productive member of society.

Still, it was nice to buy my own food and clothes. I went to a thrift store and purchased a pair of black plastic shoes that possessed all of the aesthetic appeal of orthopedic shoes but none of the comfort. They were uncomfortable, but they were mine, earned not by working for the man but by eluding the Reaper. But shoes and cheeseburger runs weren't my only expenditures, and with that first lump of money I did what any Decker would: I went to Wayne Lanes and bought my first bowling ball, the Beast.

Bowling is religion for the Deckers. Pop, my dad's dad, is in the Roanoke Bowling Hall of Fame, and in 2005 my own dad was inducted into the Augusta County Bowling Hall of Fame. I was there the night my father bowled his first perfect game—a 300—in league, and was also present when my brother did the same. My last living grandparent, Nanny, bowled well into her seventies, and is still known to hang out at the bowling alley. In short, the Deckers don't fuck around on the lanes.

Things were going along pretty well until Josh graduated from high school. His dad, whom he had not seen since he was an infant, when his parents divorced, was living in Massachusetts, and Josh left Waynesboro to live with—as well as get to know—his father. But he wasn't the only one getting chummy with his pops.

One of my dad's proudest moments came when I decided to bowl side by side with him on league night. We hadn't spent quality, organized-sporting time together since my old farm league baseball days, and with his true bowling son, Kip, away at college, I was making a damn fine substitute, and Dad and I were becoming closer than we'd been since I was a kid. "Hey," he would whisper as Mom momentarily left the room, "want to go shoot a quick game of pool before dinner?"

The basement at the Decker Compound was the hookup: big-screen TV, foosball table, dartboard, and pool table. Dad and I watched ultimate fighting, pro wrestling, and boxing, and logged many hours with my Race-to-100-Victories Eight-Ball Challenge, a series that lasted two months and can now be seen routinely on ESPN Classic. After he got to fifty-one wins, Dad shook my hand. "Good game, son."

"What are you talking about?" I said, holding up the computer printout. "It says Race *to* One Hundred, not best of."

Dad still beat me.

Most of my high school friends had evaporated, either by going off to college, landing a job, taking the next step in their life, or developing a drug habit. But I had no small-town, post–high school exit strategy. Having lived day to day for a decade, I never thought I'd wake up to find myself twenty years old and still living with my parents. The situation is not uncommon, by any means, but definitely undesirable for anyone who hasn't been rendered comfortably numb as a result of severe head trauma. In the meantime, my brother not only graduated from college, but married his junior high school, high school, and college sweetheart, Deanna.

Once again, Kip was moving forward, but my life was stuck on pause. The dilemma became painfully obvious when I ran into a blast from the past, Photon Patrick, the kid my brother body-slammed onto the sidewalk back on Crompton Road.

Patrick was moving to Charlottesville, a hip college town twenty-five miles over the mountain, and was looking for a roommate. With my monthly checks, I could swing my portion of the rent, so I figured, "Why not?" Sure, money would be tight, and I wouldn't be buying another bowling ball for $150 anytime soon, but I enjoyed the taste of peanut butter sandwiches, and the thought of getting out of Waynesboro was just as appetizing.

Charlottesville was a pretty cool place with quite a few music venues, the perfect place to launch Synthetic Division, my new band, which, like Nine Inch Nails, consisted of one person: me. At first I didn't tell my parents what I was up to, and it wasn't until Patrick and I found a place to live that I decided to speak with Mom about the move. "Well," she said, "are you sure you want to live with *Patrick*?"

Mom had always been nice to Patrick when we were growing up, but now, by coaxing me to leave, he was suddenly "the enemy." When he came over one night and played a key on her beloved piano, Mom stormed downstairs, yelled at him, and then huffed back to her room. With that, Patrick and I retreated to the basement, where I confided, "She doesn't want me to move. She still thinks I'm a fucking kid."

In some ways, Mom was right: I didn't do my own laundry, I didn't pay any bills, nor did I have any responsibilities. Mom and Dad's goal had been to see me live to my high school graduation, a goal they never thought could come true. She never imagined having to parent me past the age of eighteen, and so she never envisioned a day when I'd be ready to fly away from the nest.

Mom also worried about the place being clean enough. I'd get sick. Wouldn't have enough money. Couldn't make the rent. Would get eaten by the flesh-eating chimpanzees that preyed on the city of Charlottesville. Anything to scare me out of the move, but I wasn't budging.

This forced her to resort to desperate tactics.

"I spoke with Patrick's mom today," she said, "and she's worried about you living with him." That didn't bother me, though it seemed a bit curious. The next line is what tipped

Mom's hand. "She was wondering how Patrick would make the rent if you died."

"I hope that's the last of his concerns!" I shouted in disbelief. But her trick worked. And soon thereafter, tired of all the maneuvering, I bailed, not only on Patrick, but also on the hope of ever escaping Waynesboro. To help me settle in, I bought a dog, Goldust, borrowing the name from a professional wrestler. I took her to puppy obedience classes and walked her around the cul-de-sac and back to the Compound, but not even my new canine companion could quell my longing to escape from Waynesboro.

By discouraging the move to Charlottesville, Mom was just doing what she did best: whatever it took to keep her son alive. But, thinking back to what Kip said when we were little, I felt like I'd be better off dead than living in Waynesboro the rest of my life. And now that I was getting older, some of the rules of survival needed to shift, not just for Mom but for me, too.

One night while bowling with Dad in league, I blew an easy spare in the ninth frame that cost our team a shot at the playoffs. He didn't care—Dad was just happy that we were spending quality Decker time together—but my lousy performance on the lanes followed me home, and triggered the deeper root of my anxiety.

For so long I'd been avoiding the future like Medusa's gaze, and now I was ready to stare down adulthood. Having survived over a decade of living with my pet virus and two years with hepatitis C gave me confidence, but also made me realize that being "unabled" no longer suited my needs.

What should I do? What should I be? Better yet, what could I do, what could I be? I knew only how to live one day at a time, and my only skills seemed to be the ability to make off-the-cuff jokes and survive deadly viruses.

At age twenty, when I realized I could live to see forty, I found myself in the midst of a midlife crisis. That's when I came to an unlikely conclusion: I'd open up about the one thing I never wanted to talk about before: my pet virus.

positoid

The year I came out of my AIDS closet—1996—I decided that the World Wide Web would be a good place
to share my story, so I launched a website called "My Pet
Virus." I lifted the title from a Nirvana lyric during my brief
affair with the band (Nirvana temporarily displaced my
beloved Depeche Mode) that ended tragically when Kurt
Cobain blew his head off.

Before I created the site, I wanted to see what was out
there already, assuming there would be hundreds—if not
thousands—of websites that featured the personal stories of
my fellow positoids.

After an hour or two of searching, using keywords like
"people with AIDS," "I have AIDS," and "nude XXX," I

couldn't find anyone who was sharing their pet virus experiences.

Just as I was about to give up, I stumbled on a page posted by a Gulf War vet who'd tested positive. Happy that someone was putting it out there, I searched his posting for an e-mail address so I could drop him a line, but couldn't find one. Then I came upon this disclaimer: "I'd advise against putting your life story online, as there are some heartless people out there who will try to make your life a living hell."

I'm not so sure if it was altruism or just complete boredom that led me to want to educate others about HIV, but whatever the motivation, "a living hell" sounded pretty damn exciting. With that, I launched www.mypetvirus.com. Packed with short stories about living with HIV, it was also home to a sharp-tongued alien named Altog, who answered questions about outer space (a good way to make fun of people without having my name attached), and a list of celebrity crushes that included Katarina Witt and Drew Barrymore.

Though the virus was omnipresent, I wanted my homepage to be about me—*all* of me—and I wasn't going to let AIDS steal my thunder. In fact, I made it the butt of a lot of my jokes, because I wanted to be comfortable writing about HIV. My e-mail address was plastered all over the site, with links that read: "HIV can't be transmitted through e-mail, so drop me a line!" I wanted people to ask questions, share their stories, and have access to me. Who knows who might stumble upon the site? Maybe even Katarina Witt.

As I was learning how to navigate the Web, I started to find some people who shared not only my HIV status but the ability to laugh at themselves as well. A positoid named Misfit—a kindred geek from Topeka, Kansas—sent me a movie, *The Crippled Masters*, a little-known masterpiece that features a kung fu duo consisting of a man without legs and another without arms. (It's tricky, but the guy with legs carries the legless guy in a little baby knapsack. The guy with arms does all the punching, and the guy with legs does all the kicking.)

But the first positoid I actually befriended online was Steve Schalchlin. In his photos he was a dead ringer for Ted Danson, and he had put his diary about living with AIDS online earlier that year. "You should start one," he typed to me one night in a chatroom. "I think this public journaling stuff is going to be HUGE!"

Ironically, while I started my site to show that you could *live* with HIV, Steve had started his to document his death from AIDS. By the time I met him, however, HIV meds had turned things around, and a site that was meant to give updates on declining health to family members caught on with strangers, who had become enthralled with Steve's "return from the grave." He's still alive and writing it today at www.bonusround.com. (Unless, of course, you've stumbled upon this in some used bookstore and the year is 2062. In which case, I'm dead, too.)

Steve not only welcomed my friendship, he encouraged

me to reach out to as many people as possible. The son of a preacher, he knew the power of testifying, and his "calling" was to spread the gospel of living with AIDS without shame. When I worried that I was treating the subject of AIDS too lightly, Steve dispelled my doubts about my new positoid persona. "You have a real message of hope," he told me. "You just deliver it with laughs."

Dr. Lyman offered a message of his own. Impressed by my openness, he mailed me some issues of *Poz*, a national HIV/AIDS magazine that, I soon discovered, bums out some cat enthusiasts, who hear it as "*Paws*." He wanted me to have access to up-to-date information, but when the magazines arrived I thought, "Ugh, I really don't want to read this depressing shit." Yet soon I was sucked in by page after page of life stories, some uplifting, others not so; but everything about it was *real*, and it struck a chord. I put down the magazine, which featured a smiling positoid face on the cover, long enough to write and mail a fan letter to the editor in chief.

Now that I'd made friends who had AIDS through the computer—a personal triumph—I took it one step further: the AIDS support group. Dr. Lyman had suggested this all throughout my teen years, but at that point I wouldn't be caught dead at one of those, and found the idea of getting together with people who have one thing in common—a virus!—absurd.

But now it was a dare I made to myself; I wanted to see if I possessed the *cojones* to man up with my fellow positoids in person, so I went to Charlottesville, the site of my failed move attempt, where the nearest support-group meetings were held.

A funny thing happened on the drive over the mountain. As I was approaching my exit, a curious thought entered my mind: *Turn back while you can. What on Earth do you have in common with these people? And will they be sick?* I'm somewhat impressionable, and I really liked showing off how cool I was about my pet virus. I knew I didn't really want to hear about how terrible life with HIV was. Instead of retreating, though, I figured: *Okay, if it blows, I'll just never go back.*

As everyone introduced themselves—a formality, since they obviously knew each other—I chose my words carefully. With the time to speak drawing near, another strange thing occurred: a feeling of fear rushed through my body as I realized that I was in a room full of people with HIV *and AIDS.* I couldn't control all the thoughts in my head, but they went away quickly as members of the group—which ranged widely in age, ethnicity, and attitude—started talking about their pets, home-improvement projects gone awry, and the other day-to-day stuff. "I just bought a dog," I sheepishly said. "Oh really? What kind?"

Sure, they talked about doctor's appointments and health problems, as well as interpersonal issues concerning family and loved ones, but it wasn't scary, and soon I looked forward to the twice-a-month drive over the mountain to be in a room full of positoids.

One of the interesting dynamics at the support group was that there *was* a dividing line. Not the usual suspects of age, race, or sex, but whether you were on HIV drugs or not. At one meeting I was getting grilled on why I wouldn't start treatment, and my answer of "I don't want to" wasn't good enough. Sure, I was dragging ass from fatigue, but anything short of dying seemed better than swallowing twenty pills a day and dealing with all the side effects—diarrhea, rashes, upset stomach, numbness in legs—the meds crew always complained about. To fend off the pressure, I found a perfect job for my dormant pet virus hep C, trotting him out as my scapegoat for not going on HIV meds. "I'm not sure how the meds would affect my liver," became my go-to excuse. But I understood why the "HIV druggies" wanted me on meds: they cared. Plus, some of them remembered when meds weren't an option and wished that some of their departed friends had had the option. "If things get bad," I promised, "I'll go on the meds."

After the meetings, Bart, Anne, and I would go out for coffee and hot chocolate, which gave us a chance to get to know each other outside the group, in a less "AIDS" environment. Bart, a man in his early forties, had the occasional outburst in group, like the time he called a couple of attendees "stupid" for no apparent reason before cooling down and apologizing. But overall I thought he was funny and good-hearted. Anne, a mom, was around my age, recently diagnosed, and super-secret about her status, though she wasn't lucky enough to have hepatitis C to fall back on when she was being cornered at group about going on meds. I'd step in to defend her. So would Bart, even though he was on the pills.

Besides making new friends—online and off—I reconnected with my old friends Mark and Josh, speaking with them for the first time about HIV. I apologized for not confiding sooner, but they hadn't taken my unwillingness to speak about my pet virus in high school as a personal slight. Their main concern was that I was feeling well—which I was—and in going public I had their full support. Not that I was ever worried about that.

I felt like my life was on track: I'd put my virus to work, discovered my love for writing, and my parents, always proud of me even when I was doing nothing, were thrilled that I'd found a niche. One night after I'd been watching wrestling with Dad in the basement, the phone rang. It was around ten p.m.

"May I speak to Shawn Decker?" the mysterious voice asked.

It was Sean Strub, the founder of *Poz*.

He wanted to know if I'd be willing to go to New York to be interviewed for the magazine. I'd never been to New York before, nor had I ever been interviewed. This was *New York City*. A *national* magazine. About *AIDS*. I couldn't exactly go off spouting Altog the Alien, or some other crazy bullshit I put on my website. I needed credentials, something of consequence to say. I studied some issues of *Poz* as a refresher, but ultimately decided that I'd just have to wing it.

When I arrived at the airport, I noticed this face peeking around the corner. A rangy fellow with dark hair, Sean Strub had a very *Daily Show*–correspondent look, more Stephen Colbert than Steve Carell. Only, in person he didn't look as healthy as he did in his headshot. "It's KS," he said, aware of my gawking.

Kaposi's sarcoma. The little purplish-red splotches that appear on the skin of people with severely compromised immune systems. The Tom Hanks character got them when he got really sick in *Philadelphia* (and wasn't around much longer afterward). I'd never seen KS in person, and, assuming Sean might not be around much longer, I felt uneasy that I wouldn't have a long-lasting friend or get to know him better.

While in New York, I hung around the *Poz* office and met the staff, who kind of adopted me as a mascot. I'd been learning so much about the AIDS community—online and at support group—but being in New York showed me that there was a massive world out there, and that I had a place in it. Sean later confided in me that in the course of my visit I dispelled a lot of stereotypes that some of the staffers had about rural, small-town straight boys.

But, of course, the main reason I was there was the interview, and on a Tuesday night I met the writer, Degen Pener. He and I spoke over dinner at a somewhat fancy restaurant;

by "fancy" I mean that there aren't ten thousand of them with the same name across the country and there were table-cloths involved. I was totally out of my element. "I'm more of a grilled-cheese-sandwich kind of guy," I said. "Oh, really," Degen said as he recorded our conversation. "I haven't had one of those in years!" What a weirdo, I thought as I mispro-nounced the name of my entrée to the waiter.

Later that night Degen took me to a rock concert at a local drag club. There were blowtorches, clowns, porno movies playing on TV screens ("That's a bit much," Degen offered), and topless dancers dripping in chocolate syrup. "Cool," I said, trying to pretend that I'd been to places like this before. Degen, who sensed otherwise, responded with a smile. "In Waynesboro you only see this kind of stuff on the weekends, right?"

Stephen Gendin, the guy with the "COCKSUCKER" jacket in college, was one of the characters I met on my first trip to New York. A friend of Sean's, Stephen would dye his hair whacked-out colors—like purple, blue, and Bozo red—and then dye his little dog's tail to match. I'd never seen anyone like him before, and Stephen wasn't some aimless eccentric; he owned his own business, an HIV medications mail-order prescription service where the only requirement for em-ployment was that you were a positoid. So when he offered me a job—and Sean wanted to hire me to help rebuild and maintain the *Poz* website—I jumped at the opportunity. The only question was: Would my attempt to move once again meet with resistance from Mom? After all, people actually *die* in New York City.

Amazingly, Mom and Dad didn't give me any grief about the move, just a pat on the back and a generous infusion of cash. They trusted that since Stephen and Sean were posi-toids, too, they would look out for my health. And maybe, just maybe, Mom and Dad were looking forward to having the house to themselves for the first time since 1972.

Sean put me up in a house he owned outside the city, and I commuted into New York with his hot sister; not a bad ride at all. The only aspect of moving that made my parents ner-vous was signing a lease, something I wouldn't have to do for a few months since Sean hooked me up with a place to live.

I didn't *really* know much about computers outside of e-mailing, simple HTML, and emoticons. Plus, my knowl-edge of HIV drugs was intentionally nonexistent. I could send somebody the wrong meds and they could die, as far as I knew. Before I could even catch on, I was quickly learning that the fantasy of living in New York City was completely disconnected from reality, as were my inflated expectations of what I could do. Not only did I discover I couldn't climb Mount Everest, I couldn't even sit at a computer for eight hours a day, and working and commuting left me no energy for anything else but sleep. I was worn out, and after three and a half weeks of the city I was ready to go home.

I wanted to talk to Sean before I made my decision. I was embarrassed that I was throwing in the towel so soon, and wanted to make sure that my leaving wouldn't put him out in any way. As we sat on the porch of his house, Sean said, "Well, let me just say that *whatever* you decide, it's been a pleasure getting to know you better these last few weeks."

Around eleven o'clock that evening, my parents, who'd just gotten done packing up my room, answered the telephone. "Uh-huh," Dad said as Mom tried to figure out who was calling at such a late hour. "Yeah, I understand, that's fine, son." Buddy Decker then hung up the phone, turned to his wife, and said, *"We're fucked."*

Two days after I got home, in September, I came down with a nasty bronchial infection that lingered until just before Christmas. I was thankful that this didn't happen in New York—far away from my family—and as I recovered from the trip and dealt with the coughing spells, I retreated back into the safety of my online persona.

Despite the aborted move to New York City, 1996 was off to an incredible start— my best yet! I was dazzled by my *relevance.* I had a voice, and through the magazine everyone was going to hear it. Even though *Poz* wasn't exactly *Rolling Stone,* my friends treated me like a rock star, because magazine articles just don't happen to people from Waynesboro, a place where only one person—P. Buckley Moss—has ever gotten famous before. And that was for a series of paintings featuring bow-legged Amish folk.

When the *Poz* issue featuring my smiling face on the cover—with the title "My Pet Virus"—hit the stands I thought

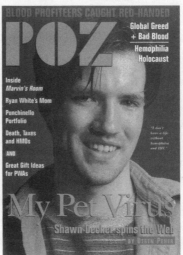

My first interview in 1996
landed me on the cover
of *Poz* magazine.

it was the coolest thing I'd ever seen or read. I know, I'm egotistical, but I saw the article as proof that I was doing something right.

In the story, Degen wrote that I was "a blossoming writer," and detailed how I gauged my health not by my T cell count but by my bowling average. There was also my getting kicked out of school, an event relayed to him by my mother that I'd apparently blocked out. As I read, the details started to slowly come back to me; damn, I thought, my life is pretty exciting. (Fun fact: Even though this issue came out in 1996, if you go to my proud mom's house you'll still find that *Poz* with me on the cover sitting out on the coffee table.)

The "blossoming writer" prophecy came true, and I started writing a column for *Poz* in which I detailed my experiences as a young, single positoid. Appropriately, the name of the column was "Positoid," a word that Sean and other positoids loved. My star was on the rise!

Steve Schalchlin was coming to Virginia to perform some songs he'd written about his experiences with AIDS, and I went to meet him in person. I have to admit, I was a little weirded out. This *was* a guy from online, so how did I really know what he would be like? And would he be hemophobic offline?

The relationship between thinbloods and gay people is often strained. Hemophiliacs resent the fact that many people associate AIDS solely with gay city folk. Homosexuals, in turn, resent the fact that "the innocent victims" get special treatment and sympathy because of the way they were infected. Hemophiliacs, in turn, are pissed that they didn't have a smile on their face when contracting the virus.

Is there a difference between receiving junked-up medication and landing a bad lay? Maybe. But the real decision-making process begins after diagnosis, because it's too late for all of us positoids once the test results are in, and in the end we're really in the same boat and face the same fearful—and sometimes painfully stupid and insensitive—reactions. So why some perpetuate that nonsense from within the community is beyond me.

After a three-hour drive to Norfolk, I arrived at Steve's hotel. I approached his room nervously and gently tapped on the door. "Positoid!" Steve's voiced overflowed with glee as the door flew open and he greeted me with a big hug. And it was comforting that—just like his online pictures—he still looked like Ted Danson to me. I took a chair by the window, and Steve sat on the bed, asking, "So how are you doing?" Before I could answer, Steve belted out, "Now, get over here already, positoid, so I can have sex with you! I promise, I won't give you AIDS or anything."

The tension officially broken, we both burst into laughs and I joined him on the bed. Steve, obviously as goofy in real life as he is online, put his arm around me and said, "I love ya, positoid." From that moment on, Steve was the gay uncle with AIDS I never had.

Soon thereafter, Steve and I were back online joking

about a terrible movie we'd each recently seen. "Hey," I posted, "why don't we do an online movie review?"

Thus was formed the Hemo2Homo Connection—two guys with AIDS, one a brash straight boy in his twenties and the other a wise gay man in his forties. No gender was safe from the sexist remarks of two friends, brought together not only by their virus but by a shared love/hate of movies as well.

I pitched the Hemo2Homo Connection to *Poz* as well as the *Advocate* but got no takers, so what should have been seen by millions of people in print as well as on television was relegated to obscurity on the Internet . . . until now.

Without further ado, I give you the Hemo2Homo Connection's best review ever, a candid look at the Oscar-winning film *The Hours*.

HEMO (SHAWN DECKER): Hey, Homo, seen any good movies lately?

HOMO (STEVE SCHALCHLIN): I saw *The Hours*. I know I'm supposed to be the gay one, but can I say that I think Julianne Moore is a goddess?

HEMO: I've had a thing for her since *Boogie Nights*. So I guess we now have three things in common—a love for movies, Julianne Moore, and AIDS. Speaking of which, what did you think of Ed Harris's portrayal of a man dying with AIDS?

HOMO: I found his performance annoying. Or maybe it was the character. "Oh, I'm so sick, so the only option I have is to jump out a window . . . Oh, I'm gay but I still love my lesbian ex-lover . . . Oh, I have AIDS, so I have no love in my life." *Bleahhh.*

HEMO: Wait a minute . . . he jumped? I thought he was pushed.

HOMO: He wasn't pushed, you thinblood. He thought he was going to have to have sex with Meryl Streep. So he did the noble thing and jumped.

HEMO: Well, regardless of how it happened we both agree that he went out the window. And I don't understand why you are mad—the AIDS guy simply follows the storied tradition of positoids in film; we always die. And if we don't die, the last scene alludes to impending death.

HOMO: Maybe he jumped because, by that time in the film, Julianne Moore was too old to have sex with?

HEMO: Julianne Moore will never be too old, my friend . . . which makes me think, shouldn't everyone with AIDS get to have protected sex with her? Color me bad, but I think that's the cure, the government knows it, and they are keeping the information top secret.

HOMO: I think you're on to something, Hemo. Sign me up for *that* experimental trial.

HEMO: Hold your wood there, buddy. This shouldn't be for everyone with AIDS. Just kids with hemophilia who were diagnosed at age 11 in 1987. I'm going to contact the Make-A-Wish Foundation and see what I can do about this.

Homo: More special treatment for you? I get it. All right, you
do that. The rest of us will have to settle for sex with Ed
Harris. But only after he gains some weight. That boy
needs a protein bar.

Hemo: Now you're making me hungry . . . not for Ed, mind
you, but for a protein bar. I'm not into sex with guys. No
way . . . not that I have anything against that, of course.

Homo: You're not fooling anyone, you know? You only got
HIV in the first place because you wanted to be around gay
men. Admit it.

Hemo: I'm just using you guys to get close to Sharon Stone.

Homo: I for one have met Sharon Stone, and she gives *great*
hugs.

Hemo: OK, you get Sharon Stone and I get Julianne Moore.
Now back to the movie. Julianne Moore's character didn't
do herself in, but she should have. That little rug rat pes-
tering your ass all day long is far worse than having AIDS.

Homo: I happen to think that you're going to try to wash
those spermies of yours and make some for yourself
someday. Just wait and see, young one. So, besides the
brat, what else bothered you about the movie?

Hemo: Well, they really should have gotten someone more
attractive to play the part of Virginia Woolf. I don't pay the
big bucks to see some homely-looking thing up there on
the picture screen. I want glamour! I want stars!

Homo: Hey, idiot, that was *Nicole Kidman in a rubber nose.*

Sheesh. If anyone should know about sticking rubber things on body parts it should be you, Hemo.

HEMO: You've got a point there. So, Homo, how do you rate *The Hours*?

HOMO: To sum up: *The Hours* is a brilliant movie, even if I didn't like Ed Harris's wacky AIDS guy. Overall it was a sensitive, brilliantly acted, wonderfully told story of heartache and isolation. On a scale of 1,000 T cells, I give it a rating of 850.

HEMO: Well done. I guess that's all for now. Until next time, I'm Hemo . . .

HOMO: And I'm Homo . . .

HEMO: And we'll see you at the movies . . .

HOMO: Or in the hospital!

One good thing about moving back home was the fact that I could get back to writing, and I took Steve's advice and started my own online journal, or "blog," as the kids call 'em today. The instant gratification came in waves of e-mail support and encouragement, and Steve and I would meet in a chatroom for our nightly jousts. When I wasn't giving him hell, I'd meet new people, chat a bit, and then send them to my website. One night, I noticed someone's name I'd seen a few times before.

SEBADOH (That's me.): Hey, that's a nice name.

MARIANA: Why does everyone say this? What's so special about "Mariana"?

In Brazil, where she is from, the name is as common as Sarah is in the United States. I wrote: "Well, Mariana, to us pie-eating, flag-waving Americans it seems exotic!" That line did the trick. Our online friendship really took off, to the point where I started getting interruptions from Steve, who saw my name listed as being in the chatroom.

STEVE: Hey, Positoid . . . you there?
SEBADOH: Go away, thickblood, I'm talking to a girl!

I spent hours a night chatting with Mariana, and the good thing about getting to know her through the computer was that it was much easier for me to type to a girl than it was to talk to a girl. This had nothing to do with being shy and everything to do with that pesky cough. The computer—and spending time on my website and in chats with Mariana—was a great way to avoid the fact that my real life, as evidenced by my showing in New York City, was starting to exhibit signs of trouble.

Since HIV is a big issue in Brazil, Mariana knew a little bit about the AIDS epidemic. The first night we met, I sent her to my website and she learned of my HIV status. I did that with everyone, because it was my "job." But Mariana didn't respond the way others did; she researched the topic online and read my entire website. I liked the attention, and she didn't hesitate to heap praise on me. She was also feisty, which matched the energy of my positoid lifestyle, if not my actual energy levels. So, one night, I had a wild idea, but I wasn't sure Mariana would be game.

SEBADOH: Want to talk on the phone?
MARIANA: . . . SURE! ☺

Her response was enthusiastic, and there may have been more than just one smiley face attached. But when the conversation happened, something was amiss; we spoke for about two minutes before the call ended awkwardly.

Back in the safety of the chatroom, I danced around the issue of the weird phone call, uncertain if I'd accidentally offended, like the first time I posted a message about her name. Thankfully, the quick dis wasn't an indication of my waning mojo; Mariana was nervous about her Brazilian accent. "You sounded great," I typed. "Really!" Mariana, hoping to be a translator someday, was self-conscious about her English—one of several languages she knew. One thing that wasn't being lost in translation was that our chats were establishing a connection that went far beyond our modem lines, and it was obvious to everyone—including my dog, Goldust—that I'd fallen in love.

Christmas in 1996 was a far cry from the first post-virus

holiday in 1987, when I almost took down Grandmother. Instead of keeping talk of my pet virus under wraps, my decision to speak out meant that AIDS was now fair game, and Mom went all out. She bought a fake white tree, lit solely with red lights, and hung little red ribbons alongside ugly, AIDS-themed ornaments. "The proceeds went to AIDS charities," Mom explained.

Mom and Dad supported not only my HIV activism, but my budding relationship with Mariana as well. The only sticking point about my love life was the monthly phone bill, which at its worst reached $500. My parents figured they'd rather help buy a plane ticket to Brazil than fork over that kind of money on long distance again, so soon I was off to spend two weeks with Mariana and her family. I'll bet my parents were thinking, "Couldn't Shawn have just found a nice girl ten miles away in Stuarts Draft?"

Mariana and her family lived in the city of Belo Horizonte, and they also owned and operated a dairy farm on the outskirts of the city. Despite my inability to milk a cow or speak more than a phrase or two of Portuguese, they accepted me with open arms. The family consisted of Papa Boliche (her dad, a bearded man whom I affectionately named "Father Bowling"), "Mama Rabbit" (she shared my Chinese horoscope, the Rabbit), and brother Dani (he was a big guy—best not to give him a cutesy nickname until I found out whether or not he approved of me).

I was at Mariana's mercy, following her around like a little lost puppy. In between seeing her cousins, aunts, uncles, and friends, we found a lot of time to talk, cuddle, and kiss, and I loved the feeling of holding Mariana in my arms.

During my two-week stay, we went out on our own for a couple of days, staying at a Brazilian UFO hotspot. But even in an area where there'd been an alarming number of sightings, I was way too busy looking at Mariana to worry about stargazing or flying saucers.

Staying with her family was a trip within a trip: her mom made sure I was fed my favorite meal, chicken fingers and rice; Dani, an obsessive fan of the Ramones, and I bonded, making up a shoot-'em-up dice game as we listened to "Blitzkrieg Bop." The approval of Papa Boliche came easy as well, and on one breezy Brazilian night at the family's farm, the two of us took an ill-advised swim in the pool after perhaps one too many drinks.

When my parents picked me up at the airport, Dad noticed the glow on my face that could only mean love. Unable to resist, he asked, "Is your little fellow happy?"

Was he ever. Mariana and I fooled around a little bit—safely, of course—at the UFO hotspot, and our chemistry offline definitely surpassed our online chats. In fact, when I got home, our postings to each other would get quite steamy.

STEVE: Shawn . . . Shawn???

Mariana decided to go to school at Mary Baldwin College,

about fifteen miles from Waynesboro, but her family was wary of their daughter traveling so far, as well as living with her boyfriend and his family. So I did what any other thin-blooded American boy would do: I proposed. Cyberly, I got down on one knee (you type the action in between two asterisks) and typed the question. *"ARE YOU SERIOUS?"* she wrote, before typing her answer, "YES," alongside an infinite row of smiley faces and exclamations points. (I sold one of my synthesizers to buy her a ring.)

Not only was our love story crossing over from cyberspace to real life, but the transition was also going to be broadcast on MTV.

A month before I proposed, I'd seen a phone number on TV for a show called *MTV News: Unfiltered,* which asked, "Do you have an interesting story?" Did I ever. I called and rambled on to their answering machine for about a minute or two about being kicked out of school, and about how I was still alive and educating people about HIV. When I hung up, I thought, "That sucked." So I called back and said, "Hey, it's the AIDS guy again . . . now here's what's *really* interesting about my life right now."

The next day I got a call back. "Tell us more about Mariana. Would she be okay with you filming and talking about the relationship?" I ran the idea by her in chat and she was excited about it. A video camera was sent to my house and I documented the saga, explaining how we met, the visa process, even the engagement. When I went back to Brazil to spend time with her family before Mariana and I returned to Virginia, I shot footage there, too.

In Waynesboro, Mariana was greeted with open arms and open paws at the Decker Compound, and she gave my chow, Goldust, a huge hug. "Goldie!" They were so cute together, and I got the sense that my dog enjoyed Mariana's rubs better than mine. Mariana got along so well with my family that she talked them into letting us get another Chow, a puppy we named Moondust. I didn't know it at the time, as we never spoke about such matters, but Mariana wanted real children someday. Not only did we not talk about growing some brats, we also weren't sure what to say when people asked us about the big wedding date; we just looked at each other and shrugged our shoulders.

Trouble between Mariana and me arose quickly, in the form of a spot developing on my side. It was shingles. I'd had an episode back in the fourth grade—two years before my HIV diagnosis—and that's when my parents knew I was a positoid. For Mariana, my second round of shingles was just as revealing. I did my best to downplay it and they cleared up with antibiotics, but when I got lab work done a month later it showed yet another dip in my T cells. Mariana cried. "It's okay," I said. In person, though, I was far less convincing in the role of healthy boyfriend.

We drove to New York City to see *The Last Session*, Steve's play about a musician dying from AIDS who wanted to record one last set of songs before offing himself. Surely this would take Mariana's mind off of my health problems. I particularly loved the lyrics of Steve's song, which included the killer line: "I'd rather be me with AIDS than to have to be you without it!" And Steve gave me a little nod, using the word "positoid" in a key scene in which the main character discloses his status to a stranger. Yes, I'd put Waynesboro on the Broadway map!

Mariana's classes were going well, and every morning she'd ride to school with Mom, who worked near the college, and I'd pick her up in the afternoon, an hour or so after I woke up. She must have been surprised by how much rest I needed, but in my mind I had enough to do what I needed to do, which was hang out with Mariana when she wasn't studying or at school. We'd go to the movies, bowl, have dinner, and occasionally fool around. Mariana wasn't freaked out by my HIV status in the bedroom, but she was definitely afraid of losing me.

On December 1, World AIDS Day, I was invited to the White House to partake in a meeting with the Clinton administration's AIDS czar, Sandra Thurman. The other participants were negatoids, kids still in high school who'd formed HIV peer education groups at their schools. I was the oldest one there at the haggard age of twenty-one.

For such an important occasion I was severely underdressed and undergroomed, having haphazardly thrown together a stray suit jacket with a puke-colored button-down shirt the day of the trip. The real problem wasn't my fashion faux pas, though; it was that, upon arriving at one of the offices outside of the White House, we were informed that Mariana wouldn't be allowed to go inside because she wasn't an American citizen. At this news her Latin temper flared up. "I'll just sit here and do nothing!" But Mariana understood that we couldn't just hop in the car and drive back to Waynesboro.

I was told beforehand that Vice President Al Gore would be making an appearance, and Mom, assuming the bragging rights, leaked word of this important invitation to the *News Virginian* in Waynesboro. Of course, in typical Mom fashion she overstated the case, and on the morning Mariana and I drove to D.C., the headlines blared: "Local AIDS Victim to Meet President!"

When Al and Tipper Gore came into the room, he lightened the mood with a couple of jokes and a cool manner that I wished he had brought to the presidential debates of 2000. Before departing to deliver meals to bedridden positoids, Al asked, "Does anyone have anything they'd like to say?"

Everyone clammed up.

"Yes," I said, taking the vice prez up on his offer. "I just want to thank you guys for putting this meeting together. I've been living with HIV since I was a kid, and I was expelled from school when I tested positive. It's nice to see that so many people here are still working hard to raise awareness."

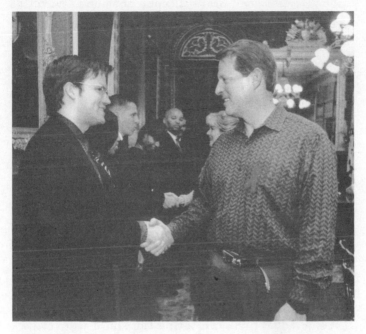

Meeting Vice President Al Gore on World AIDS Day, 1997.

My words probably weren't *quite* so polished as that, but the sentiment came across more effectively than my drab appearance. As the Gores split, one of Sandra Thurman's aides came around the large table I was seated at, and said, "Thank you *so much* for doing that."

When Mariana and I got back to Waynesboro, I read the local paper.

"AIDS Victim? . . . Clinton?" I contacted them to correct the story, explaining what really happened, while also mentioning that "AIDS victim" wasn't exactly the best way to describe a positoid like me. The next day, the headline read: "AIDS Patient Does Not See Himself as a Victim."

In her first three months of being in Virginia, it became apparent that Mariana missed her family terribly. This was the first time that she'd been outside of Brazil, and it was a big move for a twenty-year-old. So we said goodbye to Moondust and Goldust and flew down to Brazil for Christmas and New Year's.

I enjoyed my first summertime Christmas, with temperatures up near a hundred degrees. But it wasn't just the hot weather that was making me sweat. On the last night of our visit, as Mariana was trying to find the right shoes to wear with her dress for the evening, she broke down in tears. Her anguish, I realized, wasn't just about the wardrobe malfunction, and it broke my heart to think that Virginia was never going to be her home.

When we came back, things were better for a while, but I was still her only real friend in Virginia, and she still missed Brazil. I wasn't going to the support group anymore, and even though he was back in Virginia, I didn't see much of Josh, either. I spent my time with Mariana, because she needed me the most, but we didn't really know how to work out our individual issues—I was ignoring my health, and she was missing her family in Brazil—as a couple. Instead, we went to see *Titanic*—four times—at the theater.

When Mariana talked about returning home for the summer and taking the fall semester off, I understood what I'd sensed for months: her homepage wasn't going to be based out of Waynesboro for much longer. My family and I took Mariana to the airport, where we had a big, tearful goodbye. When she got home, we broke up in the same place where we'd first fallen in love: online, in our favorite chatroom.

"Hey, positoid, ya there?"

"Yes, Steve . . . I am . . ."

For the first time in months, I went back to the support group, where the response was less than supportive from my friend Bart. He usually yelled at other people, but this time he trained both barrels on me: How could I not come to group? Or call? And now I thought I could just waltz back in so easily? One of the other fellows came to my defense, arguing that living my life and giving love a shot was something that any of us would bail out for. At my car, as I was leaving, the moderator spoke to me: "I hope this doesn't change your feelings about coming to group. A lot of people here really value your presence, and Bart was way out of line."

I promised him I'd be back, but that was the last time I went.

Like most twenty-somethings, I learned a lot through trial and error. No, I couldn't work a regular nine-to-five job, but I could get on a plane and go meet a girl in Brazil, thus taking an emotional risk that few would attempt, at any age. Going from not talking about my pet virus to broadcasting it on the Internet, as well as on MTV, and writing for *Poz*— those were *my* college years, and I learned a shit ton.

a townhome at the
end of the world

J ames Lipton of TV's *Inside the Actors Studio* always asks
the stars what they would like God to say when they arrive in Heaven. Well, I doubt it happens, but if God greets
non-celebs verbally as they enter the pearly-gated community of Heaven, I'd love to hear him say: "C'mon down,
Shawn! You're the next contestant on *The Price Is Right*!"
Rows and rows of Plinko boards, Putt-Putting, and Barker's
Beauties; make that *Decker's Beauties*—Katarina Witt in her
1994 Robin Hood Olympics outfit and Julianne Moore from
Boogie Nights.

Although it wasn't a pricing game, after high school I was
offered the chance at $100,000.

In the early 1990s, thinbloods knew that blood companies had collected plasma from at-risk populations—including citizens of third-world countries with lax screening standards, gay men, and prisoners. Thus a lump-sum class-action settlement of $100,000 per infectee was negotiated. *And the Band Played On* touches on what went down, but the gist of the story is that profits were put ahead of safety; the proof was in the proportion of thinbloods infected with HIV—more than half—which showed that our bad luck wasn't so much the bleeding disorder, but our reliance on greedy corporations for our well-being.

Still, when I heard about the settlement at age eighteen, it seemed that, once again, I was being given money for nothing.

The blood companies never acknowledged that they failed to keep their products safe. So if this was a "goodwill payment," why not have a little more fun with it? The grab at $100,000 could have been less like a lawsuit and more reminiscent of, say, an episode of *Let's Make a Deal.* Think about it—a bunch of thinbloods dressed up like giant chickens, prostitutes, and breakfast food. Some would make the right call, trading in their unopened envelope for what was behind door number two, while others would go home empty-handed or, even worse, with some gimped-up livestock in tow.

My parents knew for years about all the gory details of negligence regarding my infection, and they chose not to burden their "dying son" with one more shitty aspect of a sufficiently craptastic ordeal, but when this class-action settlement offer came up, they filled me in. And I also rented *And the Band Played On*, because I was too lazy to read the book.

At the time, $100,000 seemed like quite the jackpot, and I figured if the money ever came through I could coast on it for the rest of my life. The negotiation process lasted three years, during which many would-be recipients passed away.

With Mariana gone, I decided to spend the summer with Josh and my summertime friends, who were attending James Madison University, thirty miles away. I hung out there just about every night, and as I was heading out for the evening, Dad would ask, "So what are you up to tonight, son?" "Oh, just going to get sloshed!" I was enjoying all of the social aspects of college without any of the responsibilities of schoolwork, and I was happy with the arrangement. Once again, I kicked up my feet as poor Josh trudged through his academic work.

One night, as I lay curled up on the couch in a friend's living room, fast asleep, I was awakened by someone stumbling around. I rolled over, opened my eyes, and saw one of my drinking buddies standing in front of a chair a few feet away. My glassy eyes cleared just in time to see him lift the cushion, unzip his pants, and urinate. Finished, he put the cushion down, lay down on the floor, and went back to sleep.

Dad and Mom were hoping my partying ways would subside, since hepatitis C and my liver would eventually reject this kind of a lifestyle. Also, alcohol is a known blood thinner, which may explain why I was pissing blood after a gal pal—surprisingly strong for being so diminutive in stature—picked me up and squeezed me hard in a bear hug.

All of the pissing and getting pissed aside, spending quality, altered time with my pals was *long* overdue because, otherwise, I had *nothing* to do. I didn't write a "Positoid" column about the breakup, leaving *Poz* readers sort of in the dark, considering I'd written so much about her, and the only entries in my online journal were about how well I was bowling and how many beers I drank the previous weekend. My parents probably got even more nervous when, around this time, the settlement finally went through: *I was rich, bitch!*

To celebrate, I threw a little party one weekend when my parents were out of town. I invited a hundred of my closest friends over for the blowout and, just to be safe, I covered the furniture with a protective layer of plastic. The bender is a blur, but the pictures prove that these were the best three days of my entire life. One thing I didn't anticipate was the hefty cost of restoring the Decker Compound to its pre-party splendor, and after a week all of the money was gone.

No, actually the money was used to get my own place in nearby Charlottesville, where I'd tried to move three years earlier with Photon Patrick. Now, armed with a stack of Benjamins, there was no stopping me from leaving Bow-legged Amish-land for the town that Thomas Jefferson built and Dave Matthews made famous. C'ville was like another country: vegetarians roamed the land and rich folks voted for Democrats.

Once again, Mom protested, only this time her rationale for delaying my grab at independent living was a bit more legitimate.

The place I was moving into was a bit of a fixer-upper. The old man who had owned the townhouse for over twenty years had done no renovations; the heating unit was gasping out its last breath, the green shag carpeting likely contained many rare life forms, and the whole interior decor was straight out of the late seventies.

"Why don't you wait two weeks?" Mom said. "Let your dad and me get some new carpet in there and clean the place up!"

As I was making plans to move into my new pad, I took a trip to Los Angeles to visit Steve and attend a *Poz* Life Expo, where I got to see Sean and greet readers of the magazine at my "Hug the Positoid" booth. While in California, I got a phone call from my mother: Grandmother had had a stroke, but what worried me was that Mom kept saying, "Everything will be okay," and imploring me to "Just stay out there with Steve and your friends."

The only thing Grandmother hated more than Republicans was hospitals, and she wouldn't willingly stay in one if given the choice. And more troubling than that, Mom was *downplaying* a medical event. I cut short my trip and booked the first flight home, and when I arrived at Grandmother's hospital room I learned that she couldn't speak. But her eyes were full of life. I took a deep breath and dished all about my trip out to see Sean and Steve.

Grandmother loved those guys and had met Steve when he came to perform his tunes in Charlottesville the year before. A big fan of Liberace, she decided that Steve was no slouch on the piano, either, and when we all went back to the Decker Compound after his concert she stayed up past her bedtime, talking and laughing till well past midnight. She understood what my closest positoid pals meant to me, and why it was Steve Schalchin and Sean Strub from *Poz* whom I chose as my surrogate godparents.

Grandmother read all my "Positoid" columns and kept every newspaper clipping from the town paper that mentioned me. It's funny, but when I was born she blamed herself for being a carrier of the hemophilia gene, as if she had any control over that. The fact that I not only survived but also met a Democratic vice president, Al Gore, gave Grandmother a great sense of pride, and I'm happy that some of my accomplishments allowed her to forget about that bum gene of hers.

Tired from the flight, I told Grandmother I had to go home and get some sleep, and she nodded, as if to say, "Yes, go rest! I'll see you tomorrow." That was the last cognitive moment that I shared with her, and a few weeks later she passed to spirit.

Mom was beyond a state of grieving; she was in shock. Grandmother wasn't just her mother; she was her best friend. Every day they'd smoke cigarettes together and gossip about current events and family happenings. Which presented another dilemma with the timing of my move: Would it kill me to stay home a few extra weeks? she wondered. Mom had just lost so much; did she have to "lose" her son right now, too?

This time I was the unreasonable one and, selfishly, didn't allow the family tragedy to change my plans. I gave my grandmother's eulogy, did my best to assure Mom—who knew better—that I'd still be as big a part of her life as I'd always been, and then headed across the mountain with a car full of keyboards, a computer, and a new guardian angel in my grandmother, who was now in Heaven making cafeteria-style lunches for her favorite dead liberals.

a boy, a girl, a virus

At the AIDS Services Group (ASG) in Charlottesville, some of the female employees' comments would definitely have met the criteria for sexual harassment, but I sure wasn't complaining. The innocent flirtation was a good fit for my need for affection, and I welcomed every "cute" and "if I weren't married" remark that came my way. Like my gay pals from New York, they were just trying to show me, in their own way, that I was a catch, knowing how hard I had it as a straight poz guy. After disclosing, by the way, I almost wished I *were* gay: dating would have been much easier (I wouldn't have had to fly to Brazil to meet a girl).

In Waynesboro, I could only launch my plans from the computer, but in Charlottesville I was ready for some face-to-face advocacy and education. I attended monthly board meetings of the ASG as the token guy with HIV, a role that suited me fine, as I didn't contribute much else to the meetings, which I found to be quite dull—reminiscent of sitting in a classroom. So when I got a chance to ditch one night, I got in my car and didn't look back. I was going to meet friends and see Jeanne White, Ryan White's mother, who was speaking about an hour away, at James Madison University.

I'd seen her once before with my mother, and after the program—in which she explains Ryan's legacy to a generation that was too young to know it firsthand—Mom and I took Jeanne out for ice cream at Ruby Tuesday, where the two mothers had a chance to debate treatment issues. "Well, Shawn hasn't been on HIV meds and he's doing just fine!" I just sank further into the safety of my ice cream sundae.

This time, however, I didn't tell Mom about Jeanne's visit, and at the conclusion of her presentation, I was standing in line to thank her. Since there were a lot of people at the program—about eight hundred—I had some time to kill, and I passed it joking with my friends. "How hard could it be to live with AIDS? C'mon!" "There's *no way* somebody could be kicked out of school for having AIDS." I canned the funny-guy routine when we got closer, and thanked Jeanne for coming, briefly explaining that I'd been through a lot of the same things Ryan had. When I turned to leave, a girl asked, "Are you Shawn Decker?"

She told me her name was Gwenn and that she recognized my voice from having interviewed me on the phone earlier that month for a graduate project she was working on. She had shoulder-length brown hair, attentive and engaging eyes, and an interest in HIV/AIDS, and I was a little smitten.

In addition to her graduate studies at James Madison, Gwenn was working part-time in Harrisonburg as an HIV/AIDS case manager, helping positoids keep track of their doctor's appointments and monthly bills. Since there weren't too many other twenty-three-year-olds working in the AIDS field in the middle of Virginia, I wanted to stay in touch with Gwenn, so we exchanged e-mail addresses and phone numbers, and early the following week I saw a message in my inbox: "Hey Shawn, it's Gwenn from JMU. Portions of the AIDS Quilt are going to be here, and I was wondering if you wanted to come see it?"

Wow, what a first date! Maybe she was interested in me?

A couple of years earlier, in 1996, I'd seen the AIDS Quilt in Washington, D.C. Shortly after my return from my ill-fated move to New York City, it was the last time the full set of panels were displayed together, as well as the Decker family's first AIDS picnic. Mom, Dad, Kip, and Deanna joined me, and I was kind of a bonehead—making friends with strangers and handing out cards for my website that said:

"Shawn Decker: Professional Sick Boy." Of course, being at the Quilt wasn't all fun and games. I just felt that if I could make someone smile who'd lost a loved one, then I was doing my job, and the AIDS Quilt seemed like an ideal place for positoids to connect.

At that time I didn't have any friends' names to look for, which may account for my lack of gravity. But I did notice a few panels for Ryan White and Pedro Zamora from MTV's *The Real World*. I had watched the show that season, taking in everything Pedro said, never thinking I'd ever put my virus out in the public domain. Though I only knew them through their education work, those guys were, and are, my positoid heroes.

Before revisiting panels of the Quilt with Gwenn, I visited my aunt Mary in Waynesboro, who learned how to cut hair on Kip and me when we were kids. She'd gotten really good over the years, and hooked me up with a new Charlottesville look: gone was the floppy hair. Now I wore short hair and a hint of sideburns. When I met Gwenn in Harrisonburg, at a local eatery, I was hoping to sweep her off her feet, but she mentioned her long-term, long-distance boyfriend, Nathan. Very classy of her, I thought, but still a bummer.

Gwenn and I went to see the Quilt panels and then returned to the eatery to say our goodbyes. But instead of getting out of my car and leaving, Gwenn stayed and we talked for what seemed like an hour, before going inside to continue our discussion over ice cream.

While Gwenn was an undergrad at Wittenberg University in Ohio, a young woman came to speak to her Delta Gamma sorority about living with HIV. The woman had been infected by her boyfriend, and aside from being positive, she wasn't all that much different from Gwenn or her friends, which made Gwenn wonder why young people weren't more interested in learning about—and sharing—ways to prevent HIV transmission. She manned booths at high school health fairs, showing teenagers how to properly use condoms, and I was impressed because, unlike me, she chose to get involved with AIDS, not the other way around.

The next week, I invited Gwenn to an AIDS event at a high school, where, as the lone representative of sexually transmitted infections, I was speaking on a panel with teen parents who were regretful that boners had transformed them from horny teenagers into clueless parents. Afterward, Gwenn and I went to dinner at the same Ruby Tuesday where my mom and Jeanne White had debated. Behind us sat a mother and her two unruly kids, and although technically we weren't on a date, Gwenn was about to utter the words that would make my heart flutter. With a nod to the table behind ours, she said, "I have no maternal instincts whatsoever."

Apparently the interest was starting to go both ways. She went to my website and read the very first "Positoid" column I had written, entitled "Sex & the Single Positoid," a spirited little piece about all the great things I have to offer the ladies that don't lead to changing diapers. Rather than a guy with

HIV, I was a self-described "willing young stud capable of fulfilling one's every fantasy." Upon reading the column, Gwenn shot me an e-mail: "Hmmmm . . . I've got a few fantasies of my own."

Whoa.

Even after the saucy comment and my retort—an inquiry into said fantasies—our flirtation remained platonic. She was dating another guy, plain and simple. Far be it from me to complicate matters by revealing my crush.

As Gwenn and I continued to rack up the late nights together—watching TV and talking about our lives and views—we soon found ourselves cuddling up at her place, my arm around her as she nestled into my chest. Soon we were having innocent sleepovers, bouncing back from my place to hers. I didn't mind the one-hour drive; really, it seemed like a luxury that Gwenn was in the same country.

Her best friend, Jason, took notice.

After hearing story after story about this new character in her life, Jason challenged Gwenn to acknowledge why she was willing to drive an hour to see me every other night and was increasingly blowing off Nathan. "Something's going on," he told her. "You really like this guy, Gwenn!"

Even though Nathan lived about four hours away, what frightened me was the fact that he was a six-foot-seven jock who had played basketball in college. Not only that, Nathan was studying to become a doctor, which meant he also possessed the technical knowledge of how to hurt someone. As my feelings for Gwenn continued to grow, I was convinced that the natural conclusion of our relationship would be my being beaten to a bloody pulp.

Over Thanksgiving I pined for Gwenn when she went to visit her family in Cleveland, and then again at Christmas. On New Year's Eve, Gwenn and I were together, and as we were leaving my house—going God knows where—I remember wanting to plant a kiss on her as she was putting on her shoes, looking up at me with a smile that seemed to say, "I love you," a thousand times over.

Though I knew that Gwenn's long-distance love was on life support, I wasn't happy to be tripping all over the wires, and one morning I explained how I felt. I'd be around for her as a friend if that was what she wanted. But I needed to know, one way or the other: Is that *all* she wanted from me? Gwenn was uncomfortable with being confronted, but she understood. Jason's take on matters was that Gwenn was in love with the idea of Nathan, but not the person.

Emotionally we were already attached, but the dilemma Gwenn faced was understandable: Stay with a decent relationship that's on autopilot, or take off on a new one to destinations unknown? Nathan was a kind, handsome, and very tall guy with a promising future as a doctor; I was a hemophiliac who had just gotten his hair dyed blue, walking toward an uncertain future in discount orthopedic shoes. At twenty-three most girls would dream of having a guy like Nathan, but I was hoping that Gwenn would defy logic by choosing the "AIDS patient" over the dashing doctor.

About a week later I was having drinks with friends at my place, which didn't have much decor. There was artwork, made by my friends of varying degrees of artistic ability, haphazardly thumbtacked up on the wall. For "mood lighting" I had a strand of Christmas lights hung above the couch, and it always threatened to fall on the unsuspecting head of a guest.

To my delight, there was a knock at the door and it was an unexpected guest: Gwenn.

Her hair was pinned back and she had on a modest amount of makeup, just enough to accentuate her natural beauty: her soft brown hair, kissable lips, and hazel eyes. Gwenn looked even more beautiful than usual, and not because I was tipsy, but because I wasn't expecting to see her for at least a week, which was one of the reasons I was tipsy in the first place. "I hope you don't mind me crashing the party," she said.

No, I sure didn't.

The party continued, and later that night two of my friends crashed out in the living room. Gwenn and I went upstairs to get her settled in the spare bedroom, where, as we were lying together on the bed, I put my arm around her, my chest to her back. And that's when it happened: we kissed. And then kissed some more. I'd waited so long, as had she, and now all of our bottled-up emotions were spilling over, which gave me the answer I was looking for. This *was* a relationship, and thanks to the friendship we'd already built— not to mention that first kiss—Gwenn and I were off to a great start.

At the time, my "chance" meeting with Gwenn hadn't seemed strange. But now? I have to think that other forces were at work.

How else can you explain that I—the very picture of responsibility—skipped a board meeting to be at Jeanne White's talk? (Okay, I'm anything *but* . . .) And that Gwenn skipped—with permission—a class so she could attend? And what about the odds of her standing behind me? There were lots of students waiting around afterward. It's not exactly Power Ball odds, but it makes me wonder: Was Ryan White up there in the rafters, pulling strings from above in an effort to hook a fellow thinblood up?

I like to think so, because if anyone knows how tough it can be for a guy like me to land a chick, it's Ryan.

eleven

beauty & the beast

A glaze of Krispy Kreme goodness dangled from the corner of my face, but by then, Gwenn and I were in that phase of utter amorous obsession where nothing could come between us, not even bad eating habits. Of course, these days, I can't get away with having food on my face, even when I say, "I'm saving that for later!"

As we were chowing on doughnuts that night, I'd discover that, just like myself—in the past—Gwenn was harboring a secret.

"So, what are you doing this weekend?"

"Well, nothing Friday," Gwenn said, "but Saturday I'm busy."

"Oh, what are you up to?"

"Nothing really," she said, looking away. "Just this . . . *thing*."

My curiosity was piqued, as I thought we'd already plumbed our deepest, darkest secrets. Perhaps Gwenn was a contract hit woman for the government, or a high-society call girl? Whatever was happening on Saturday, I wanted a piece of the action.

"All right," she said, buckling under the pressure. "I'm doing a pageant. There. I said it."

Before that night at Miss Blue Ridge Mountains, I would never have guessed I'd become an expert in pageantry. Never wear clear plastic shoes (you'll look like a pole dancer), never snatch the microphone from the host onstage (makes you look a little bull-dykish), and always smile. As weak as your smile is, *always smile.* And use whitening toothpaste. The audience can't tell if your teeth are crooked, but yellow comes across loud and not-so-clear.

Living most of my life in Waynesboro, I'd never been to a beauty pageant that I hadn't accidentally stumbled upon in a parking lot at Rose's department store. Luckily for Gwenn, this pageant was taking place inside of a high school. I bought a program book for five dollars, and within the pages I found my first picture of Gwenn, not to mention some handy information. Age: twenty-three. Platform: AIDS. Talent: monologue. Really, outside of those three things, what else do you need to know about a human being?

For the uninformed, the "platform" is a social issue one

cares about, and is discussed during the private-interview phase of judging. Most pageant girls just crap out something, like caring for animals or volunteering, but I knew firsthand that Gwenn *cared* about AIDS. And if she didn't, well, that was okay, because she cared about *me*.

The lights were lowered, and the spotlight hit the stage as the contestants walked out to introduce themselves. The music was up-tempo, like something from a Gap commercial, and the girls marched up to a microphone and screamed their names into it. Some of them might have been deaf, like that Miss America from several years ago, but if it was just a ploy to get people psyched, it worked; I was pumped up and primed for some serious female-on-female combat.

Seated down in front was one of the contestants' mothers. I overheard the woman bragging that her daughter was going to take the crown. "Yeah, right," I thought. "Gwenn is going to hand that girl her overgrown ass." I was starting to get a little catty, but Gwenn was ruling. Her onstage interview was smart and sassy. Her swimsuit was smokin'. Her talent . . .

A girl can squeeze herself into a tutu and slide around like a puppy on a hardwood floor and she'll still get more talent points than Maya Angelou reading a poem. There is a pecking order when it comes to pageant talent, and for pageant judges the monologue is the bottom of the barrel; they hear you talk in interview; they want to see some pizzazz on that stage.

Well, Gwenn doesn't sing, and Gwenn doesn't dance. Most girls who have this dilemma wear a nice dress, wheel out the piano, and bang out a few chords, but even then you run the risk of going up against some girl who's played piano since she was four. Gwenn did a dramatic monologue about a woman who has just learned that she has HIV. Stunned were the elderly women in the crowd, expecting another baton-twirling routine to "The Star-Spangled Banner."

Despite her inability to do soft-shoe, Gwenn was by far the brightest star on that stage. The verdict loomed, and I clutched my program book in anticipation. Fourth runner-up. No Gwenn. Third runner-up. No Gwenn. Second, first . . . you got it, still no Gwenn. Finally, the winner was announced and the bragging woman stood up and let out a primal victory scream.

If my seat weren't attached to the floor, I'd have belted her with it.

Emotionally worn out from the two hours of competition, I went to congratulate Gwenn. "Hey, good job . . ." I said before being cut off. "Let's get the fuck out of here," she whispered.

This was the first time I saw the fiery side of Gwenn, which I have since come to know, love, and fear. In vain I attempted to be a calming presence. "Oh, don't worry about it," I offered.

"This is total bullshit."

"Uh . . ." I backtracked.

"Total. Bull. *Shit.*"

Sequins, flowers, and fury surrounded me in that high school auditorium. Camera flashes snapped, well-wishers mobbed contestants, and I tried, unsuccessfully, to console Gwenn, whose family lived in Ohio, meaning that she had no obligation to hang around and play nice. She fumed like an impending chemical explosion, and we left before she choked the judges with the sash of the newly anointed Miss Blue Ridge Mountains.

We drove back to her apartment in Harrisonburg and I realized that Gwenn would never be crowned Miss Congeniality. No, her mission was far greater: to become Miss Virginia.

The only way to get into junior high schools to talk about AIDS in Virginia is to walk in in high heels, a suit, and a crown, and Gwenn was determined to do just that. And the only way to get the chance is to win a local—like Miss Blue Ridge Mountains—and then go on to Roanoke in June to compete with over twenty other local pageant winners for the state crown. Gwenn knew she needed guidance, so she enlisted the services of a close friend, supporter, and pageant expert: Guru.

Guru, who has worked closely with numerous former Miss Virginias and pageant queens across the country, knows all and sees all on the pageant stage. Thanks to Gwenn's sincere interest in her platform issue, he took an interest in her when she first started competing in Virginia, a year before I met her.

I didn't know it, but Miss America is really a scholarship

program for women, and winning these pageants helps contestants pay off student loans and negate the cost of higher education. Of course, some girls put more into the competition—in pricey gowns and shoes—than they'll ever get back, and, sad to say, most of those clothes are terrible.

Guru was perfect, because his frugal eye could find outfits for Gwenn that looked great but didn't cost a lot. And he understood every facet of competition—including platform—and ways to stand out.

"Gwenn," Guru said, "if your platform issue is HIV/AIDS, then why don't you talk about your relationship with Shawn?"

Gwenn was aghast at the suggestion. Pimping out her boyfriend for a chance at pageant glory? Unethical. "Gwenn," Guru continued, "you see all those other girls doing it, and their stories are boring and stupid. My God, one girl talked about the death of her grandmother's dog. Now, *this* is different."

I thought Guru's plan was a masterstroke, and I didn't mind being whored out for educational purposes, especially if Gwenn would benefit. Even though it was just beginning, I encouraged Gwenn to tell our story. "Seriously," I said, "just see what happens."

Not only did Guru overhaul Gwenn's interview technique, he revamped her talent, the part of the contest that was holding her back. If Gwenn could fix that, as well as add the personal story, then she would have a one-two punch

that could rack up enough points to get her to Roanoke. With
a front-row seat to Gwenn's training program, I had a real
crash course in pageantry via Guru's mystical knowledge of
the inner workings of the pageant system. Wanting to help, I
sprinkled some humor to add optimum impact to Gwenn's
once depressing, now comedic monologue. Thus "Trixie" was
born, a loudmouthed, southern bride wannabe wearing huge
white platform shoes, a wedding dress, and 1950s cat-eyed
glasses. People were going to laugh before Trixie even opened
her mouth, and Guru knew that this was one monologue that
would score big.

Armed with newfound talent and poise, Gwenn was ready
for Miss Powhatan. But a couple of days before the competition, she called me and said, "Shawn, I need to talk to you
about something."

Those words are never good. Either someone is pregnant
(impossible) or someone wants to break up (impossible?).
Maybe she was having second thoughts about Nathan, or
worse. Fully clenched, I prepared for the worst.

"It's about the pageant," she said. "Would you mind not
attending?"

"No problem," I said, relieved that it was my presence *at
the pageant*—not in her life—that made her apprehensive.
"Thank you, thank you, thank you," she said.

Miss Powhatan was an hour away, and Gwenn promised
she would come to my place after it was over. In the meantime,
I got a call from her best friend, Jason. "How'd she do?" he

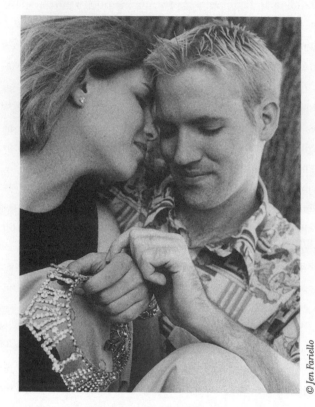

© Jen Fariello

**Falling in love with Gwenn,
and pageants.**

asked. "Well, I haven't heard back yet. But it's late, it should be over by now." Jason knew Gwenn's pageant obsession better than I did—she'd competed in over ten without winning a single one. As Jason continued to speculate on the results, I heard the door open. Gwenn was on her way upstairs, and as she rounded the corner I screamed like a girl into the phone. *"She's wearing a crown! She's wearing a crown!"*

Gwenn was the new Miss Powhatan! And she was going to Roanoke!

Instead of worrying about my weight issues—a result of a recent loss of appetite—Guru was putting pressure on Gwenn to get in the gym and tone up. "You need some sun and a little time on the treadmill," Guru instructed, thinking that a little of the "AIDS look" I sported might garner her more points in swimsuit competition.

Not that Gwenn was out of shape. It's just that these girls train like soldiers for Miss Virginia, and Guru knew that every point counted. One local pageant director, he told us, actually makes her winner stay at her house for two months before the Miss Virginia contest. Her home is equipped with a swimming pool, and the lady sits in a folding chair all day smoking cigarettes and yelling, "Two more laps! Two more laps!"

The big stage at the Roanoke Civic Center was a far cry from the high school auditoriums where Gwenn had met defeat so many times before, but she wasn't the only one out to score points that weekend; I was meeting her mom, Beverly, for the first time.

Gwenn grew up in a suburb of Cleveland, having been adopted at two months old by loving, albeit incompatible, parents. Though they divorced shortly thereafter, Gwenn never faced a shortage of family, and as the only "kid" around, she was doted on by loving grandparents and a barrage of aunts and monosyllabically named uncles—Uncle Rob, Uncle Tom, Uncle Jim, Uncle Bob, Uncle Ron—who, in addition to their three-lettered names, had one thing in common: a great love for Gwenn.

Naturally, Beverly was very concerned about HIV transmission. Gwenn assured her mom that there was little risk of her getting infected, particularly since we are both educators and had a full understanding of HIV prevention. The next fear was: What would happen if I got sick?

At the time, I was still having trouble with food, but in a way so was Bev. Her problem was the opposite: she was overweight and used a wheelchair to get around, which made traveling to Virginia a real pain for her. But there she was, anyway, and as with any good mom, there was no way Bev was missing this event.

Since Bev had worked in a doctor's office, I was hoping she'd empathize with my medical situation, and when I saw that we were laughing at the same jokes, I knew I'd won her over and that we'd get along fine. Now it was up to Gwenn to win over the pageant judges and crush the dreams of twenty-eight other hopefuls.

It was the final night of Miss Virginia, and the moment of truth had come: the ten finalists were about to be announced, and they would go on to compete on the live statewide telecast, broadcast immediately after the announcement. The rest of the girls, who didn't make the ten? They would be forced to stick around and perform lame song-and-dance routines. I was hopeful about Gwenn's chances, because she had held her own during the two days of preliminary competition. Even so, I couldn't forget the scars of Miss Blue Ridge Mountains.

"The next Top Ten Finalist is . . . *Gwenn Barringer, Miss Powhatan!*"

Gwenn paused, stunned, and the girl beside her had to confirm it was really her name that had been called. The audience of 1,500 erupted. Gwenn wasn't just the darling of her family and friends—she was now a strong crowd favorite. As she walked to the front of the stage, a stunning vision of beauty and aplomb, I cheered, presenting a less-than-impressive physical specimen. Like most of the girls up there, I too had lost a lot of weight in the preceding months. But my weight loss wasn't to squeeze into a swimsuit; it was the result of my pet virus—not some pageant coach—wearing me down.

During the Top Ten talent, I could hardly wait for Gwenn. There were some old standard pageants songs, a Disney song, a tap dance, but nothing quite like Trixie, who hiked up her wedding dress and lamented the fact that she doesn't get free stuff as a single woman, punctuating her plea with an angry "My trailer needs stuff!"

Another big moment came during Gwenn's onstage interview, when she announced that the issue of HIV/AIDS work was now personal for her, because her boyfriend was HIV positive. In all the dress-up, show-pony fun that is a pageant, this moment truly resonated, and during intermission several people came up to me and said, "I'm so glad she said that." Gwenn's public declaration was a simple statement that normalized people with AIDS and gave comfort to those in the audience who had also dealt with the epidemic.

But sadly, Gwenn wasn't crowned.

Bev was happy to see Gwenn in action, but she wasn't the only mother in attendance; Mom was there as well, and she told Gwenn, "You blew your chances at the crown when you talked about Shawn!" Sure, she may have lost Miss Virginia, but Gwenn sure won over Pam Decker, who learned that her son's new girlfriend was carrying a big set of balls under that sleek black evening gown.

Whenever Gwenn and I look through our photo album, it's incredible to see the difference between the two of us in the pictures from that night. We're both smiling widely, and she's beautiful as can be, but my face is thin, my eyes tired;

not the skeletal look that one usually has when they go from
170 to 140 pounds, but a decidedly frailer version of myself.
As much as I wanted Gwenn to win that year, I was very for-
tunate that she did not, because I needed her at home, not
gallivanting around as Miss Virginia or Miss America.

Weeks after the pageant, Gwenn moved in with me, and
our townhouse most certainly needed stuff: a new washer
and dryer, dishwasher, painting, carpeting. Anything you
can think of. I still had money left over from the settlement,
and a government payment from the Ricky Ray Relief Fund
provided another $100,000 because of governmental negli-
gence in the blood-industry crisis. Plus, Mom and Dad
chipped in, relieved that I was finally cleaning the place up.
Of course, the one appliance that needed the most renova-
tion was Gwenn's live-in boyfriend, and the next step in our
relationship wasn't as simple as just playing house.

twelve

just say . . . oh, no!

I am ready for the cure, I am sick of being sick.

—Lauren Hoffman

I can't wait until I'm thirty-three," I said to my grandfather one day after receiving a stern talking-to from him. I was six years old, and though I don't recall exactly what I did wrong, I do remember that my grandfather chased me down the street after I made an unsuccessful escape attempt.

"Thirty-three? Why thirty-three?" Grandad asked, catching his breath.

"Because then you'll be dead!"

It wasn't a kind thing to say, but the old fellow laughed it off and even proudly shared the story with family and friends. In my defense, the math held up: I'm thirty, and Grandad's been dead for a few years now. What I didn't expect when I busted Grandad's chops that day was that I might not make it to thirty-three.

Nineteen ninety-nine wasn't the party Prince promised back in the eighties; it wasn't even the party I'd enjoyed the summer before, when I was getting sloshed with my friends. At twenty-three, I was sipping on cans of Ensure, the nutritional supplement drink senior citizens take to keep their weight up. Though I'd developed a taste for the chocolate beverage, sometimes it was tough to get through the full eight ounces, and my stomach was so finicky I could barely enjoy a bowl of my beloved cereal, Lucky Charms.

The problem was that my immune system was collapsing as my virus was multiplying and eating up most of my T cells. Not only was my appetite affected, but my energy levels were at an all-time low, and for the better part of four months I gradually got worse as I waited to get better, perhaps by the power of the magic marshmallows floating around in my discolored bowl of milk.

There were many reasons for the decision to remain HIV drug–free, the least of which was that so much of my positoid identity had been built around *not* being on meds. I couldn't lift weights, nor could I brag about how many women I'd slept with in my life, but at cocktail parties no one could hold a candle to "I've been living with HIV for over ten years and I've *never* been on antiretroviral drugs!" And a lifetime—extended or not—of taking toxic pills didn't appeal to me.

Perhaps my hard-luck experiences with hemophilia treatments tempered my stalwart resistance, as it was the wonders of modern medicine that landed me with my pet virus to begin with. Plus, I recalled the pressure to take the early HIV drug, AZT, in 1988. Taken alone, AZT proved to be quite nasty, and my decision not to go on that early treatment was a good one.

Being tired was something I'd been dealing with on and off for years, and though it was sort of kicking my ass, HIV wasn't as scary as the thought of the uncharted territory of AIDS meds and the unnerving prospect of no longer being the master of my own domain. Yes, maybe my strategy to go head-to-head with the virus without meds wasn't the smartest, but at least my success or failure wasn't dependent on the effectiveness of a pill. There had to be another way to get better, I told myself.

I bought a green bike at the mall, figuring I'd exercise the AIDS off. Then it was vitamins and ginkgo biloba, but they did nothing to help my energy, or my lab results, either. I'd seen friends like Sean and Steve benefit from the HIV drugs, but that didn't change my attitude; they were sick and they *needed* them. In my eyes, my weight loss wasn't so much *AIDS*, just a glimpse into the life of the waif model.

Steve didn't sugarcoat his concerns. "You *are* sick, positoid. You need to deal with this *now*," he urged.

The seed of my antidrug ideal may have been planted before I even knew I was a positoid, back in the fourth grade, when a friend of mine brought a bag of oregano and flour to school, pretending it was pot and cocaine.

He'd meticulously removed the blade from his father's razor, but his fine attention to detail was not rewarded with extra-credit points. Instead, we all got a visit from a cop. Unimpressed with our little game of *Miami Vice*, the man in blue warned us about the realities of drug use and peer pressure, though, interestingly, the horrors of prison sex were not touched on. "Drugs will take over your life," he said, "and then ruin your life." Each student swore never to dance with Mr. Brownstone, and if you overlook a massive head-lice outbreak, I was successful in staying clean through the remainder of my elementary school tenure.

Dr. Lyman noticed my drastic decline and thirty-pound weight loss, but our banter remained the same as always. "You should think about HIV drugs," he'd say. "I will," I replied. And I didn't lie. I thought about them—and I thought they sucked. But Dr. Lyman had a gateway drug he thought I might be interested in. "Have you ever heard of Marinol?"

Marinol was synthetic THC, basically pot in a pill. When I read about it, my curiosity was piqued. Ads in *Poz* showed empty muffin wrappers covered with a few crumbs. I longed for the days when I could polish off a snack like that without having to take breaks between bites, but I'd never smoked pot and was skeptical about getting the munchies. Would this really work?

Around the time that Gwenn was preparing for Miss Virginia, I started on Marinol, figuring it was worth a shot. Being me, I opted for a half-dose of 2.5 milligrams, and after

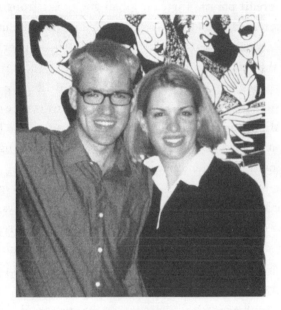

Gwenn and me in 1999, the year I got sick.

taking my first pill, Gwenn and I went out to eat to test the results. "It's probably way too soon to have any effect," she reasoned, but I figured what the hell and ordered chicken fingers with french fries. When the plate came, it was filled to capacity, but instead of viewing the dish with my usual indifference, I glared at the chicken as if it were a wanton lover, beckoning to me: *"Take me, I'm yours."* I put the food away like a Japanese hot-dog-eating champ, and when the waiter arrived with the check, I asked, "Can I get a chocolate milkshake?"

My stomach felt satisfied for the first time in three months. As happy as I was, I was a little bummed that I didn't feel stoned. Oh, well. I was content, recalling that Ensure had been a terrible substitute for a real milkshake. "I'm driving," Gwenn said as she took the keys.

There was a light drizzle that night, and as we approached the first stoplight on the way home, I felt like my life was in danger. Was it my realization that if I didn't change my aversion to HIV meds my health would only continue to deteriorate over time? No, it was that Gwenn was driving like a bat out of hell, tearing up the road in an obvious attempt to kill me.

"Slow down! You're sliding all over the road!" I said, more than a bit jittery.

"I'm not sliding anywhere," Gwenn said calmly, obviously aware of what was going on, then added, "And you, my dear, are *completely high.*"

Another person who noticed my frailty was her best friend, Jason.

For Gwenn's twenty-fourth birthday I decided to surprise her with a trip to L.A. to see Jason, so I booked the flight, worked it out with him behind the scenes, and off we went. "That's the sweetest thing anyone's ever done for me!" It was the first birthday, and I didn't want to blow it, no matter how sick I was.

After Gwenn and I arrived, the three of us went to the mall to look around. Now, I was already having trouble hanging with Gwenn in the Charlottesville mall; I'd poop out after about thirty minutes. And that place is pretty quaint. So when we entered the Beverly Center, I knew I was in *way* over my head. After a half an hour, I asked Jason and Gwenn, "Do you guys mind taking me back to the apartment?" I was done. I blamed the long flight and crashed out on his couch as they drove back to the mall.

But Jason, who had never seen me before, knew better. He said to Gwenn, "You didn't tell me he was *that* sick!" Gwenn did not think too much about the comment at the time, because she believed me when I said I would get better soon. "I know my body," I said.

And so did she.

Like any new couple madly in love, Gwenn and I were having our fair share of sex. The best thing about being with Gwenn was that we'd spoken about safe sex long before we found ourselves doing the various things that sex entails.

And she knew that condoms, when used correctly, don't break or malfunction. So the sex was plentiful, stress-free, safe, and fun.

The cloak of romance prevented either of us from fully confronting what was going on, which is why it took Gwenn a while to realize that such a stud, capable of fulfilling one's every fantasy, could be . . . *sick?*

A unique side effect of Marinol was my increased interest in shopping. Boredom, as much as lack of energy, was at the heart of my terrible shop ethic, but with me on "M-bombs," as I called them, I was willing to try on a pair of pants. Gwenn took advantage of this, and took the opportunity to deep-six my stupid-looking orthopedic shoes. "Try these on," she said in the shoe store. I put the pair on and couldn't believe how good they felt. It was almost orgasmic. "It's like I'm walking in giant pillows!" I said, pacing around the store excitedly. By that point, a pair of comfortable shoes wasn't the only thing I was long overdue for.

Considering my T cell decline, I should have gotten the AIDS diagnosis years before, but there was never a big dramatic moment at Dr. Lyman's where he said, "Oh my God, you now have AIDS!" Maybe he knew the word would cause unnecessary harm to someone who thought "HIV" stood for "Horseshit, I'm vibrant!"

The belated announcement that AIDS had arrived came shortly after our visit with Jason, and it came from an unlikely source: Guru.

Well, not exactly Guru, but he did suggest that in order to create more buzz about Gwenn's participation in the Miss Virginia pageant, we should contact the local papers. "The media would *love* you guys," Guru stated. He mentioned a free local arts-and-entertainment weekly, and I sent the people there an e-mail about Gwenn and me. When they did an article, the cover of the weekly featured a black-and-white photo of me looking kind of serious, above the title "Love & Death."

Death?

The writer, Eric Hoover, was my age, and we got along well during the interviews—one over lunch, and one at my townhouse. The piece spanned from my childhood to Gwenn's quest for the crown. Eric also spoke with my *Poz* pal Sean Strub, who said that I was "on the leading edge—nay, the bleeding edge—of the culture," referring to my educational technique. My pet virus, of course, got some ink, too.

". . . Despite his positoid philosophy, there are days when he gets down. In his shirt pocket is a box of cough drops. He has a nagging hack that just won't go away. Some days, he has no energy to do anything besides lie around. A brand-new green bicycle sits in his kitchen—he has only ridden it once."

The bits about my health struck a nerve, because Eric was right. I was sick, and I guess I needed to read it in a newspaper for it to sink in. But I was far from dying . . . wasn't I?

The thought of dying from an AIDS-related illness really hadn't crossed my mind in many years, not since my HIV diagnosis at age eleven, when it led me down a dark aisle at the video rental store: the Horror Section. I'd seen my fair share of slasher flicks up to this point, but with death on my horizon, I was drawn to *Return of the Living Dead.*

When I learned that I was HIV positive back in 1987, people with AIDS were viewed as monsters, not unlike the decaying flesh-eaters of the *Dead* films. It's one of the reasons Rock Hudson was shunned in Hollywood and Liberace's name was dragged through the mud. At that time, I was so worried about looking visibly sick. So it's funny that, when I finally was in that situation, *I* was the only one who couldn't see it, even though I walked through malls like a zombie, slowly dragging my feet along until I found a bench to rest on.

Shortly after the publication of the "Love & Death" article, Gwenn got a job in Charlottesville, at the AIDS Service Organization.

The hours were flexible and the executive director, a friend named Kelly Eplee, had an interest in HIV advocacy dating back to when a cousin, sick from AIDS, spent his final days with Kelly and his wife. He had also been a Southern Baptist minister, a reminder that religion and compassion for people with AIDS can go hand in hand. Upon hiring Gwenn, Kelly explained, "I didn't offer her the job because she was your girlfriend. She really was the most qualified person."

Just as in Harrisonburg, Gwenn was now a case manager working with positoids, only this time, when she got off work she was coming home to AIDS *and* her boyfriend, all wrapped up in one package with a little red bow.

On good days I'd be on the couch; on bad days I'd still be upstairs in bed. Either way, I was usually hanging on every word of Oprah's "Remember Your Spirit" segment—a sure sign of impending death.

Though I wore a brave face and told Gwenn I'd get better, I was acknowledging in my music that the wheels of my well-oiled positoid machine were coming off. I was working on a CD called *Tainted Goods*, and the songs were about topics like memory loss, which I was experiencing then. (Unfortunately, I can't give any examples because I don't remember losing my memory.) In one song, I sang, "I just want to relapse," an ode to the joys of being sick, which provides the benefit of no responsibilities. Optimism did creep in, though, with Josh and Steve contributing to the last song on *Tainted Goods*, an ambling instrumental that wouldn't sound out of place in a *Stars Wars* cabana scene. Another pal, Barton Lidice Benes, contributed the cover art.

Barton is famous for collecting awe-inspiring pop-culture relics such as Sylvester Stallone's urine (scooped from a urinal) and Hitler's spoon. Fans send the things in, and Barton, once he's confident of their authenticity, displays them. But he's probably just as well known for using his own positoid blood in his work. When I told him about *Tainted Goods*, Barton was happy to donate the image of one of his pieces: a green squirt gun attached to a syringe, shooting his blood.

Synthetic Division made it into the newspaper article, too, and Eric—whom I became friends with—turned me on to a local band called Bella Morte (translation: beautiful death). I picked up their CD, and they were *good*. I couldn't believe that this kind of music was being created right here in my new hometown, and Bella Morte ran a local gothic/electronic music night—The Dawning—from the basement of a sushi bar called The Tokyo Rose. I paid Gopal Metro, the bass player, a visit, hoping I could get a gig.

With his tattered clothing and many piercings, some through his bottom lip, Gopal reminded me of those punk-rockers from *Return of the Living Dead*, and, not surprisingly, he shared my love for the film. He worked near the University of Virginia, selling piercing paraphernalia, hair dye, and witty, liberal-leaning bumper stickers at a now defunct novelty store called Coyote. His physical appearance, though a little alarming at first, was accompanied by a gentle demeanor. "Hey, what can I do for you?"

After chatting, I finally got around to the real purpose for my visit. I whipped out one of my CDs and explained Barton's art. Gopal's eyes widened. "That's so rad!" He opened the case, took out the disc, and asked, "Mind if I give it a listen?" The music started. "Is that you singing?" "Yeah," I said. "It's all me, actually." "Rad." My songs didn't match up to Bella Morte's, and once the six-song disc finished, I wasn't sure if I'd be granted access to The Dawning. "My new songs are better," I said, a bit desperate. But Gopal nodded, handed me the disc, and asked, "So, when can you play?"

I scheduled the gig two months in advance. This would give me enough time to finish those new songs and deal with the nagging little issue of my pet virus, which now had rabies, as evidenced by a T cell count now below 50, a pitiful number. My viral load was through the roof, too, and Dr. Lyman had retired. I'd actually outlasted the old fellow.

My new physician, Dr. Greg Townsend, shared the general assessment of my physical state. Unlike Dr. Lyman, however, Dr. Greg didn't have anything to judge me on except for the lab results and my emaciated physical presence. "You are at serious risk for opportunistic infections," said Dr. Greg, an affable man with a hearty laugh—though on this day he was all business. "Let's start you on HIV meds. Today." Dr. Greg gave me the list of potential side effects as well as the number of pills I'd take per day and I, of course, chose the combination with the fewest pills, as the concept of going on meds was hard enough to swallow. "I'll make sure you remember to take your pills," Gwenn said, holding my hand.

I knew this moment was coming, so a week before the appointment with Dr. Greg I'd planned a trip to Myrtle Beach, South Carolina, to celebrate my twenty-fourth birthday.

The last time I was at the beach, my brother helped me celebrate turning twenty-one by taking me to a strip club with his friends. I ended my big night by throwing up in a garden. Three years later I was returning to Myrtle Beach for a different kind of celebration: my last birthday as an AIDS-drug-free man. Ready for the one last hurrah, I invited Josh and his girlfriend, Jenny, to join Gwenn and me for the four-day summer vacation. And they promised to take me to a strip club.

This wasn't my first road trip with Gwenn: five months before, when she was still living in Harrisonburg, and a month after our first kiss, we drove to New York City to celebrate *Poz*'s fifth-anniversary issue, which brought together eight former cover-story subjects for a group photo shoot. I got to stand beside Rebekka Armstrong, the former *Playboy* Playmate who tested positive for HIV. If you read my blurb in the magazine, it's full of promise: a new girlfriend and a hopeful outlook for the future. But the night we got back to Virginia, I stayed at Gwenn's place, so tired and sick from the flu that I didn't leave for a week. If that first road trip was any indication, the odds of me making it to the ten-year *Poz* anniversary shoot were getting slimmer, just like me.

The trip to New York marked the beginning of my decline. I was hoping the trip to Myrtle Beach would be the beginning of my recovery.

Despite my frailty, my friends didn't take too much pity on me, and on the eve of my twenty-fourth birthday, I was outvoted: we were going to a sushi bar. Even with my trusty Marinol, I wasn't sure if I'd find something to eat, but I didn't protest; I was with three people I loved. (And they promised that a miniature golf competition would precede the pole-dancers.)

I've never been adventurous with my palate, and my childhood diet of grilled cheese, hamburgers, fries, and shakes has stayed intact. And so, surrounded by Asian decor and menu items I didn't recognize, I turned to Gwenn for guidance. "This is *kind of* like a french fry," she said. But at that moment it wasn't the unfamiliar smell of raw fish that caused my stomach to stir, it was the familiar presence that entered the restaurant.

"Just go talk to him," Gwenn said as I shuffled the rice around my plate.

"Are you sure? I don't want to seem weird or anything," I said as I looked over my shoulder again to make sure that the object of my anxiety had not yet left the premises.

"You *are* weird," Gwenn said. "So just go over there already."

At the bar sat Ric Flair, who was having a drink with his son, David, who was about my age and sported the same shorthaired, bleach-blond look as me; we could have been brothers. In his 2004 book, *To Be the Man*, Ric Flair talks about this particular time as being one of the worst of his career. He was depressed, working for a company that no longer respected his contributions to the industry. I didn't realize this then, but his career was paralleling my sad state of health.

"Uh, excuse me, Mr. Flair," I tepidly said, my voice cracking; I was more nervous talking to the former wrestling champion than I was addressing the vice president of the United States. "I met you twelve years ago. I'd just tested positive for HIV." Flair instantly gave me his undivided attention, listening intently as I continued. "Taking the time for pictures meant a lot to me, as well as to my family. I was too young to say much back then, so I just wanted to say thanks." He returned the compliment with a firm handshake, turning the tables of gratitude by saying, "No, thank *you*."

I floated back to my table, thinking back to when I met Flair the first time. I was a twelve-year-old kid dealing with an enormous burden of fear and uncertainty, ignoring my health concerns as well as I could. The strategy worked for a while. But now, if I actually wanted to enjoy life, I'd have to face HIV and what it was doing to my body. I thought: *What would Ric Flair do?* Well, he'd fight back, and I decided that when I got home, that's exactly what I'd do.

I repeated, verbatim, the impromptu speech I'd delivered to Flair a few seconds earlier. "Too much?" I asked my friends. "No," Gwenn said. "I'm sure he likes to hear those kind of things. It's probably quite refreshing." Josh added, "No, man, you *should* have said," adopting a mock southern accent and raising the pitch of his voice a few notches, "'*Remember that time you hit that guy with the chair on his head? . . .*'" We all shared a laugh, and I excused myself to the bathroom before we made our exit. As I washed my hands, I looked in the mirror and laughed again, thrilled that I had been overruled by people I loved and we weren't in some overcrowded burger joint.

When we left the restaurant, Jenny and Gwenn burst into giggles. "What's going on?" I asked, hoping there wasn't food dangling from my mouth, and I checked my zipper, too, just to be sure. Turns out that while I was in the bathroom, Flair noticed Gwenn, and, falsely assuming that she was a wrestling fan as well, looked her over and asked, "How are *you*?" "Fine," she responded. As we were getting into the car, Gwenn asked Jenny, "Is it just me, or was Ric Flair kind of checking me out?" Jenny, still giggling, concurred: "He *definitely* was."

Ric Flair thought my girlfriend was hot. I'd finally arrived.

But more important than the Nature Boy's blessing, I came to terms with the benefits of starting treatment. Maybe things wouldn't change so much. I owed it to Gwenn to give it a shot.

After six weeks on the pills, Dr. Greg called to give me the results.

"Your viral load is 864," he said.

Quick lesson: The "viral load" is a measure of how much the virus is humping itself in your bloodstream. The more it "reproduces," the worse you feel and the more susceptible you are to getting sick. I was so tired and groggy when I started meds because my viral load was up around 800,000.

Every time I got tested in the previous months, the number would double. So when Greg said "864," I assumed he meant 864,000.

"No," Greg corrected. "Not eight hundred and sixty-four *thousand* . . . It's 8-6-4, period!"

The meds were working, and my energy levels were sky-rocketing.

I was coming to terms with life on meds; I personalized my pillbox with plastic ninjas, ordering them to guard my HIV meds, the bottles of which I kept in a Day of the Dead (the Mexican holiday, not the movie) treasure box, adorned with skulls and bones. My favorite pill, Marinol, held a special place in that box, and it mellowed me out a bit.

Until the night I totally freaked out.

When my prescription ran out, Dr. Greg refilled the Marinol at the normal dosage level—5-milligram pills—and after taking my first one, it hit me: aliens weren't invading Earth someday, they were already here. Now! The catalyst for this line of reasoning was a *People* magazine cover story, titled "HOLLYWOOD: How Thin Is Too Thin?" As I gazed at Calista Flockhart's skinny arms, big eyes, and long face, my UFO fascination suddenly horrified me. And now that I was wise to them, did the aliens—who were using fame and acting as a cover—know I was onto them?

Gwenn was out, and that's when the premonitions of my own death started. I called a friend, repeating the time of my death over and over again. "Seven forty-one . . . It's tonight! If I die at this time, save this message and play it for people!" That friend never returned my calls again, and in a twist of irony, he went on to write about aliens, er, celebrities, for *Us Weekly*.

To thwart Flockhart and the rest of her species, I jumped in the shower at seven thirty-eight, assuming that White Rain shampoo would protect me from their subliminal death rays. When Gwenn got home, I toned down the story so she wouldn't think I was crazy, but when she said, "You're kind of scaring me," as she backed away, I realized that it might be a good idea to give the "M-bombs" a rest.

It was a balancing act of sorts, because while the HIV meds gave me energy, they upset my stomach. Marinol helped the food go down, but the meds made sure that, on occasion, it would come back up. When I threw up at The Tokyo Rose the night of my first performance as Synthetic Division, however, I couldn't really blame it on the HIV medications: I was nervous as hell.

Before the show, Gwenn helped by carrying most of my equipment out to the car as I carried a bag of cords. When we got to the club, Gopal helped her bring in the equipment, and he and I set everything up for the sound check. But once it was go time, I would be on my own.

Thirty minutes before showtime, the three of us were sitting in a booth upstairs, enjoying some appetizers, when I realized I'd soon be performing in front of a roomful of strangers in black eyeliner. Just like Eminem in *8 Mile*, I ran to the bathroom and hurled. "Don't worry," Gopal said as I slumped back in my seat. "If you mess up, nobody will even know. They've never heard your songs before!"

He had a point.

Playing the twenty-five-minute set was a rush, and as I pushed buttons and attempted to remember my own lyrics, I noticed the bobbing mohawk of Bella Morte's lead singer, Andy, and a few corseted booties shaking. After the final note of my set, the crowd clapped and cheered so loud that the patrons upstairs could hear the ovation. I was an underground hit! And, let's face it, nothing gives you more credibility in the goth world than actually being in the process of dying.

Though the songs were about death, it looked like the Grim Reaper wasn't playing backup keytar in Synthetic Division after all. My energy levels were vastly improved, I felt better and the lab results were showing that the medications were working. I started to wonder if my body could take over now, because the diarrhea and the vomiting were taxing after ten months. Plus, I'd purchased enough rolls of Charmin to toilet-paper the Statue of Liberty five times over. I told Gwenn and Dr. Greg that I needed a break. "How about a switch?" the doctor asked. But I dashed his hopes. I was adamant.

The drug holiday, as positoids call them, was short-lived. Turned out my pet virus was an antiretroviral drug junkie, and if he didn't get his fix, *I* was the one who suffered. Within a month my T cells dropped, so I started on a different combination of drugs, which, no surprise, made me suffer in a different way.

I wasn't dealing with physical side effects this time; now it was a cloudy mental state and far-out dreams, like the time I woke up and saw a tall Mexican guy in my closet. As I rubbed my eyes, fully awake, he stood there with his impressive mustache, wearing a poncho and staring as he slowly disappeared from the feet up, like Captain Kirk being beamed up by Scottie. (Note to Trekkies: Forgive me if Kirk disappears from head to toe, and not vice versa.)

The medications weren't just affecting my dream state. I wasn't talking about how I was feeling to Gwenn; I couldn't go off my medications, I didn't see the point in complaining about them. So I spared her the details of my throbbing headaches and wandering thoughts because things could be a lot worse: I could be in another country or financial situation with no access to medications, or I could have gotten sick ten years earlier and died.

Even so, I needed to make yet another change. So I started on a week-on, week-off cycling of treatment with Dr. Greg's blessing, and it worked. Half the drugs meant half the side effects, and my T cells spiked to above 400, a level not seen in me since Madonna was actually still a virgin. Better yet, it helped clear my head to a point where I could have free-flowing conversations with Gwenn again, without feeling paranoid and crazy.

As I was adjusting to life on meds and keeping Gwenn in the loop—even when I was feeling loopy—we decided to take our relationship public, beyond the scope of the stage of Miss Virginia and the local newspaper: we wanted to speak publicly about living together with my pet virus.

thirteen

q & aids

So please don't ask me again, please don't ask her again
It's okay, you didn't know we have a long time waiting.

—ENGINE DOWN

Since HIV prevention work is what caused us to meet, it seemed natural to put our love story—in its entirety—out there, and just one year after our relationship began, Gwenn and I started answering questions about our sex life. "Oh my God," Gwenn said, peering out from behind the curtain that separated us from 1,300 students at the University of Kansas. "This is crazy!"

The first time we spoke together was for a class at James Madison University, where Gwenn had attended graduate school. There were about fifty students present, and the discussion went pretty well. *Much* better than when I spoke alone. I'd rather watch a monkey hump a football than view tapes of me speaking solo, PG (pre-Gwenn).

That's what led us to the hot tub.

"Let's rehearse what we're going to say," Gwenn said as she batted away my pawing hands. "You go first."

"Okay," I said, clearing my throat. "Uh, my name is Shawn, and I have HIV. . . ."

"No, that sucks. Don't say that!"

"What?"

"Would you want to hear that as the first thing at a presentation?"

"Well . . ."

"Start over."

The hot-tub boot camp on our back patio continued well into the night. My life was being hacked apart like a Thanksgiving Day turkey, but Gwenn's words rang true; my storytelling ability needed a serious polish. And, really, who cared how many toys I got as a result of my trips to the hospital as a kid or who my favorite member of Depeche Mode was?

Once we were satisfied with the skeleton of our presentation, Gwenn and I searched online for a speaker's bureau and came upon CAMPUSPEAK. As we scrolled the roster Gwenn noticed one of her heroes, Miss America 1998, Kate Shindle, whose platform was AIDS. Like Gwenn, Kate wasn't your typical pageant girl, and she advocated condom use and clean-needle-exchange programs. They also represented Steve, the Homo to my Hemo. If there could be an ideal home for our would-be speaking career, this seemed it.

Our approach was simple: talk about how we both got involved in HIV prevention, how we met, and then open it up
to questions and encourage queries into our personal life.
"Let's not allow people to submit questions anonymously," I
offered.

To see how it would work, Gwenn contacted the Delta
Gamma chapter at the University of Virginia and asked the
young woman representing them: "Want my boyfriend and
me to come speak on World AIDS Day?" They said yes.

Now, before I go any further, I have to get this off my
chest. Who in the hell decided that December 1 would be
World AIDS Day? I'd like to meet the guy who thought, "Hey,
let's fill in that void between Thanksgiving and Christmas—
when nothing is going on—with something that screams holiday cheer . . . Hey, I got it!"

We also spoke to teenagers at a church—I have no idea
how that happened—and it went well, too. It was too bad that
we decided to videotape our talk at Piedmont, the local community college, because midway through, the nerves and the
meds became a lethal combo, and during question and answers I asked a question of my own. "Where's the bathroom?" When no one responded immediately, I shouted,
"Now!" I barely made it in time.

After losing lunch, I rinsed my mouth out, washed my
hands, and returned to finish the talk. "That's life with HIV,"
I explained.

We sent the tape to CAMPUSPEAK in 2000, and they sent us a contract. That fall, we began our lives as speakers, answering questions about how we keep Gwenn safe from HIV in a program we call "A Boy, a Girl, a Virus, and the Relationship That Happened Anyway."

Usually things are pretty tame. People laugh at my jokes and respond favorably to our candor. But one evening in New Jersey, as I was explaining how Gwenn and I use condoms to keep her safe, a voice bellowed from the back of the dark theater.

"Liar!"

"Excuse me?" I responded.

"LIAR!!!"

The voice boomed once again, twice as loud. I was eager to find out what prompted such a biblical outburst. The young woman stood up, put her hand on her hip, and asked, "You mean to tell me that you've never felt the inside of a woman?"

Well, not with my dick. Since I couldn't say that, I explained that, in terms of having penetrative sex without a condom, no, I have not felt the inside of a woman.

"Okay," the student continued, this time addressing Gwenn. "But what if your man is all hard and rolls over in bed and you don't have a condom around?"

Gwenn explained that it is not the duty of a woman to satisfy a guy every time he gets a boner, but if the boner in question is in need of servicing and there isn't a condom around, don't use a plastic bag—drugstores are open twenty-four hours a day. Get in the car, or phone a friend who you expect has condoms *and* owes you a favor.

The most interesting questions often aren't asked in a public forum, as most people are not as comfortable putting it all out there as that young lady in New Jersey was. This makes e-mail the safest route for some to express their concerns without feeling embarrassed.

I'm happy to answer just about any question, even the stupid ones. And, yes, there *are* stupid questions. (A recent e-mail asked: "What if you are watching a movie and something comes out in your underwear?" Answer: The HIV burns through the underwear, seeks out Gwenn's vagina, and infects her with my deadly virus.) But I know HIV is confusing, and this is my job and passion, so I really don't mind. In the past five years, the most common questions Gwenn and I have been asked, thankfully, aren't so stupid. They are:

Q: Gwenn, what does your mom think?

A: In the beginning, my mother wasn't thrilled; she had concerns about transmission of the virus, and had never knowingly met someone who was HIV positive. Since Shawn and I had been friends for a few months before we started dating, she knew about him. What made the biggest impact was when she met Shawn in person; she really loved his sense of humor and saw that he made me very happy. And that's what she really cared about.

Q: Can you have kids?

A: Shawn and I can have kids; the question should be "Do we want to?" If we ever get to the point where that's a consideration, there is a process called "sperm washing," where the sperm is separated from the semen. HIV is in the semen and not the sperm, and following this process the sperm is tested for the virus just in case, before in vitro fertilization. It's been proven effective—as well as expensive—but if Shawn and I ever wanted kids we'd probably adopt. At this point, however, we don't even have a houseplant.

Q: Shawn, are you afraid of dying?

A: Not really, because I don't think that physical death is the end, and that provides a level of comfort. Of course, I could be wrong, and if I am, then I won't really know when the time comes, will I?

A lot of folks say they are cool with dying, and during a flight home from one of our talks, I got proof of my own stoicism about death. A few moments after we lifted off during a thunderstorm, there was a loud boom and the plane shook. The flight attendants scrambled about the plane in a frenzied state, and the pilot immediately came over the speaker asking passengers if they saw where we'd been hit. Calmly, I turned to Gwenn and said, "It's been a good life."

In the beginning, I was afraid of dying from AIDS, because the process sounded horrible and I was just a kid.
But now I accept my death—in whatever form it takes—as
part of this journey. I think so many people are so afraid of
death that they don't allow themselves to enjoy life, and I
find that sad.

Q: What's your prognosis, and how do you feel?

A: When I was diagnosed they gave me two years to live. Tops.
Twenty years later, I'm doing well. So no one really knows
what the future holds. I could live out the rest of my life
just fine. And the funny thing is that these days when I go
to get lab work done, I'm more worried about my choles-
terol than I am my T cell count.

As for symptoms of HIV, I'm not even sure. Fatigue is
something I've always dealt with, so I just make sure to
pace myself and not bite off more than I can chew. Plus, I
love naps, and can take one on a moment's notice. Today,
I'm bothered mostly with the side effects of the medication, which can cause fatigue as well, and sometimes it's
confusing: What's because of the virus and what's because
of the medication inside my body that's fighting the virus?

Q: Gwenn, do you think about HIV every time you and Shawn
have sex?

A: No. If I thought about HIV in the moment, then sex
wouldn't be very fun, would it? Shawn and I are aware of
what makes condoms effective, and using them correctly
is automatic for us. The condom is simply a part of sex,

because we can't say, "Just this once," and not use one, like some couples do.

Q: Gwenn, how often do you get tested?

A: In my case, testing isn't the primary concern; it's keeping me safe in the relationship that takes precedence. The first time I got tested, Shawn and I were worried, even though we'd always been safe. It really showed how scary the test is, and why some people who feel they are at risk will not take it. In many ways, there is just as much stigma surrounding the HIV test as there is in the virus itself, but I think everyone should know their status. If you're positive, do your best to keep the virus to yourself. If you're negative, do your best to stay that way. The only way to find out your status is to get tested.

Q: Gwenn, do you ever fear a condom will break?

A: In the beginning I did, yes. But it wasn't all-consuming. From my work as a case manager, I knew there were postexposure HIV medications. Nurses and health-care professionals have access to drugs that reduce the risk of HIV transmission in case of a needle stick or some other accidental exposure to blood.

Not that I feel like Shawn and I would ever need that. We've been together since 1999 without one condom breaking, so I don't really worry or even think about it failing.

Q: Shawn, does it bum you out that you have to use a condom?

A: Some guys get defensive. Not me. When I see a condom come out, it's not a downer—quite the opposite. I know I'm doing something right if there's a condom in Gwenn's hand, because I'm about to get lucky. And that makes me happy.

not without my condom!

I will stand up and fight for the condom at every opportunity. We're buddies; he's got my sack. I've got his back. That's why I was angered when I came across this troubling quote in *Newsweek* magazine:

> "I would not ever recommend that one of my patients have sex with someone with HIV with a condom. Because I know the statistics. They break. They slip. What we've done is not told the whole truth about condoms."
>
> —DR. TOM COBURN, CO-CHAIR OF THE PRESIDENTIAL ADVISORY COUNCIL ON HIV/AIDS

Regretfully, I must concede that Tommy is right about one thing: We haven't told the whole truth about condoms. They are not 100 percent effective. But what Tommy doesn't tell you is that human error accounts for the small percentage of failures: forgetting to pinch the tip, not holding the base of the condom when withdrawing from the vagina (or wherever else the penis has been hanging out), or using a condom whose package has been punctured.

Abstinence, for all of its political safety, has a few flaws of its own. During an eight-year study on "Virgin Promises," teens who swore to remain un-bootylicious until marriage were more likely to postpone vaginal intercourse. The bad news? I guess you could say they found a couple of loopholes in the Promise to work with. They were engaging in unprotected oral and anal sex to appease their beckoning hormones.

Yes, I think everyone should wait to have sex until they are ready. But I do feel like, regardless of their initial plans, everyone should have the information needed to use condoms effectively. And I believe that information should be taught in school.

Magic Johnson doesn't agree.

I felt a connection to Magic because in 1991, when he announced on television that he was HIV positive, I was sitting in my tenth-grade homeroom class, the only kid at school who knew exactly what he was going through. By going pub-lic he opened up an important dialogue, and for many people his infection took heterosexual HIV transmission out of the realm of myth. So when the sports legend was speaking at the University of Virginia, across town, I had to be there.

Gwenn and I plopped down the ten dollars to spend an "Evening with Magic." Most of the eight hundred students were there to find out how his jump shot had held up and whether or not he was still friendly with Larry Bird, but I had other questions on my mind. Here we both were, a decade later and healthy, and I wanted to find out what he thought about the lack of HIV education in the ten years since he was diagnosed. After a few students asked some questions about basketball, I stepped up to the microphone.

"Do you feel like public schools have started to slack off on teaching young people about HIV/AIDS and safe sex?"

"Uh," Magic stuttered, "I think that's something that parents should talk about at home with their kids."

Though I was disappointed, I can't say I was totally shocked by his answer. At that time, Magic had not publicly discussed his HIV diagnosis in many years. During his short-lived talk show he didn't bring it up. In his defense, I couldn't imagine being famous and having to announce your HIV status to the world just days after finding out the news yourself, and Magic's public profile probably didn't allow him the opportunity to process the information.

Gwenn's question was next.

"I'm in a relationship with someone who is HIV positive, and I was wondering how your wife handles it?"

Magic replied that he and his wife hadn't discussed the virus in seven years. Gwenn was speechless, a rare thing. Then Magic shifted gears and turned the conversation toward Gwenn and me. "Take care of your man," he said, looking over at me and smiling. "Rub his head. Cook him some dinner. Just take care of him. Love him."

The sentiment was kind, and I have to admit I was moved. Magic seemed genuine, but the emotional three-pointer wasn't quite what Gwenn was shooting for. To make matters worse, I later tried to get some domestic mileage out of that moment using Magic's words. Anytime Gwenn was cold with me, I'd remind her, "Be nice, baby. Remember what Magic said? So get in the kitchen and fix me something to eat, woman!" That tactic was permanently benched when Gwenn got a frying pan from the cupboard and threatened to level my head with it.

Our speaking really took off in the first year, and Gwenn didn't have time to continue her job at ASG as a case manager. Luckily, there was still a lot of "blood money" left, and my parents were still helping us out—"Hey, we put your brother through college," they said. "We can afford to help you, too." I guess instead of house payments, Gwenn and I had AIDS drugs payments, the meds and my insurance costing us a good chunk of change per month, so their help was definitely appreciated.

One of the stranger aspects of speaking publicly about our sex life is that, as a result, Gwenn and I started having less sex. Nothing kills the libido like having to answer questions about sex—and AIDS—over and over again. And if I'd known that speaking about sex would have inadvertently caused us to have less of it, then I'd have let those poor college students fend for themselves.

One of the best things about public speaking is that, by traveling, you get to visit friends who live all around the country. People you wouldn't normally see. One of the worst things about speaking is that sometimes you visit with people you normally wouldn't want to see.

Gwenn and I were speaking to a class at the University of Virginia in town, and twenty minutes into our talk the door opens and one of Gwenn's former clients rolls in, literally, in a wheelchair. Okay, the more the merrier, I thought. And then I realized it was my former friend Bart, the guy who ran me out of the support group.

After Gwenn and I finished our introductions and disclosed that, yes, we do have sex, I opened it up for question-and-answer. Things were going well, and then Bart raised his hand. Since he was right up front, I had to call on him. "Shawn," he said, *"where have you been?"*

Going reclusive on Bart had nothing to do with adjusting

to meds, and I was annoyed that he showed up. After responding to him, Gwenn and I moved on to some non-stupid questions.

Ten minutes later, Bart raised his hand again. "When can *I* speak?"

Gwenn and I don't enjoy panel discussions, because you never know what someone else's agenda might be, and the teacher of the class surprised us by inviting other speakers. The class, two hours long, was only thirty minutes in, but I wrapped up anyway and let Bart and Len—another positoid—take the floor.

When I said I was a shitty speaker before I met Gwenn, it was nothing compared with Bart's ten-minute story about diarrhea and how he once accidentally shit into a fan and blew feces all over himself and his bedroom. But the shit really hit the fan when Bart claimed that he was infected while using a condom that *didn't* break: Immaculate infection!

Len was better, but not by much, and after telling his story about being infected via unsafe sex, he opened the floor to questions. But no one—not even Bart—raised a hand. That's because you have to create a comfort zone when a difficult topic like AIDS is being discussed, particularly if you want it to be interactive. And after hearing Bart's and Len's confusing speeches and confused views, nobody really knew what to ask. So Len berated the students. "Now seriously, you *have* to have questions for us. We're here to talk to you about having AIDS. We're all men up here." Then he paused and corrected himself, looking at me. "Well, not Shawn, he got it through blood transfusions."

It takes more than a lack of shyness and a microphone to be a speaker, and sometimes people ride Gwenn and me for getting paid to talk about our personal lives. But when you consider that most people have a mortal fear of public speaking, and that the majority of those with no public-speaking phobias suck at it, you can see why this *is* a job. One that, despite my use of humor, I take very seriously.

Really, it's not so much the *speaking* that I consider the work, it's the traveling—the delays, the uncomfortable hotel beds, and the difficulty of finding somewhere, besides McDonald's, to eat. I'll never forget the time when I was flying cross-country and the largest guy on the flight moved to the seat beside mine because his headphone jack wouldn't work and he was watching the movie, *Patch Adams*. Then he guffawed at all of Robin Williams's shenanigans while spilling food on me for the next two hours.

Personally, I don't feel guilty about pimping my virus, because meds are expensive and the virus has freeloaded off its host for too long. And even with my speaking, my parents *still* help support me financially, handing me unmarked envelopes under the table whenever we have dinner. (They love *The Sopranos*.)

At a conference a few years ago, I noticed a young female college student talking to Gwenn before our program. I hung back, because I could see that the girl was speaking in a low voice and looked apprehensive. Later I learned that her boyfriend was HIV positive, too. After the talk, the same girl came up to Gwenn and walked out of the room with us. But now she was smiling and laughing, because—finally—she wasn't alone.

fifteen

my big fat today
show wedding

Gwenn and I have our own separate bedrooms. Sure, we can cuddle up and fall asleep together anytime we like; it's just not a necessity to end each day in close contact with each other. The truth is, we *really* like to sleep.

Recently I heard one of those dubious statistical studies that claimed that seventy-seven percent of couples in the United States sleep in the same bed. Unlike most couples, Gwenn and I can sacrifice a little unconscious proximity due to the fact that we spend an unusual number of our waking hours together—staying up all night watching *Six Feet Under* and *The Gilmore Girls* on DVD, roaming around town during the day and traveling together for work. Most couples don't spend as much time together as we do, and I guess that's why we don't feel the need to listen to one another snore and fart all night.

One question I wasn't ready for when I started speaking publicly was whether or not Gwenn and I would get married. Over time we adjusted, and when the question came Gwenn would just put her hand on her chin, look at me, and pile on. "... *Well?*"

In truth, Gwenn didn't really care, because she knew neither of us was going anywhere in the foreseeable future. My health was fine; her weekly fan letters to Justin Timberlake remained unanswered; life was good. In all seriousness, we just weren't interested, and—as with our weak parental instincts—Gwenn and I agreed that holy matrimony wasn't the end-all, be-all of a relationship. That's why I was completely blindsided when Gwenn asked me to marry her.

We were staying at Sean's bed-and-breakfast in Milford, Pennsylvania, the home of the bloody American flag that was used to cradle Abraham Lincoln's head when John Wilkes Booth shot him (a tourist attraction for presidential historians and thinbloods alike). As we sat on the porch, Gwenn, visited perhaps by the ghost of Booth, fired away with *the question.* "Will you marry me?"

I should have known it was coming. For months Gwenn had been reading wedding magazines. "I'm just looking at the pictures!" she said, defensively. This must be the female equivalent of a guy saying "I subscribe to *Playboy* for the articles."

Not that I was against marrying Gwenn. We'd built an in-credible life together over the course of three years, and I really couldn't wait to see what else was in store for us. I just thought we'd agreed to spare ourselves the flawed concept of the American wedding, in which someone invariably gets their feelings hurt, their expectations unmet, all the things I've arranged my life to avoid.

I said yes. But one condition would have to be met: she'd obey *me*. No, actually, the only law of our marriage was that nothing could change with the things we held most dear: my Monday-night pool league, her shoe addiction, and the night-owl hours that our relationship was built on.

After the engagement, Gwenn and I continued to get asked *the question* at our talks, and Gwenn still did the hand-on-chin thing, and I played along. And since we hadn't told our parents we were engaged, I didn't feel bad about keeping college students in the dark. After one talk, we spoke to a nice kid in a wheelchair who wrote for the college paper. Off the record, we confided that we actually were engaged, but reiterated that it was a secret. Two weeks later, we went on-line and discovered that his article blew the lid off our en-gagement. Fortunately, our parents weren't so Web savvy in 2002.

Realizing that you can never, ever trust a journalist—even if he's disabled—Gwenn and I coasted along for a year with our secret engagement, until our friends Michael and Tom brought up the topic of marriage.

"The *Today* Show Wedding is accepting applications!"

Michael and I met when he noticed my profile in the Death Issue of *Poz*—in particular, what I wanted written on my tombstone resonated with him. ("I'm coming back to eat your brain.") Since he was a townie, too, Michael sent me an e-mail and I met him for lunch. His partner, Tom, was from Ohio, just like Gwenn, and the four of us sometimes rented movies and watched *Sex and the City* together. We trusted their opinion, but . . . a *Today* show wedding?

The grand prize was everything a couple could need or want for a wedding: the favors, the clothes, the dress, the cake. To apply, you simply write and tell them all about yourselves, and each year more than two thousand couples apply for the freebie. From that pool of hopefuls, *Today* narrows the field down to four sets of lovebirds. Then the viewers vote on who wins, and the chosen pair gleefully appear on the show every Wednesday morning during the three months leading up to their wedding, which takes place live on the show.

This sounded exciting to me, but Gwenn wasn't into the idea of getting married on television. I embraced the concept, and thought it would be a great way to teach people that positoids can have normal relationships, too. Gwenn just thought that we had already put enough of our personal life out there as it was, so we didn't apply.

When the winner was chosen, I willed myself out of bed to

see what all the fuss was about, as our own baby, little TiVo, had yet to become an integral part of the household.

The groom had character, but he appeared uncomfortable. I found myself hollering at the TV, "C'mon, pal, loosen up!" The guy was blowing it, particularly when he was asked what his favorite band was. The reluctant groom replied, "Uh . . . I don't really have a favorite." Fuck! I'm sure all of his friends who were in bands would have loved having their name mentioned to a live audience of millions. Who did this schmuck beat out to win the contest?

That's when it dawned on me: Gwenn and I could *really* take this thing.

I saw myself in the groom's wedding shoes. Instead of sucking the energy out of the studio, I'd trade one-liners with Matt Lauer as Katie Couric giggled like a smitten, naughty schoolgirl. Each Wednesday after the show, Matt and I would do lunch, making fun of the terrible gown the *Today* audience had picked for Gwenn that day. "She *fucking hates* veils," I'd confide. As we became closer friends, Matt and I would start to discuss more serious topics—God, death, the true meaning of life—and after the honeymoon, I'd write a memoir about my inspirational friendship that would become the best-selling *Wednesdays with Lauer*.

"*Today* Throws a Wedding" was growing on me like a cancer: What would happen if Gwenn and I applied?

I convinced my bride-to-be that applying for this fell

within our job description as educators, because if it worked out, we'd educate millions of people without even trying. Gwenn was swayed, but she didn't think we had a chance and figured that once the rejection came in, I'd finally shut up about Matt Lauer already.

Aside from *Today*, another thing eating away at me was the fact that I hadn't *properly* proposed to Gwenn. Not that I have anything against the girl asking the guy—or the guy asking the guy for that matter. When it comes to marriage, I say anything goes. Still, I couldn't believe I didn't see her matrimony resolve weakening with each viewing of yet another television show about weddings. To rectify that lack of perception, I sprung into action.

While Gwenn was in Los Angeles to visit Jason, I ordered a vintage 1940s ring, one nobody lost any limbs over. Since it's so hard to surprise her, I thought about hiring someone in L.A. to put on a mask—with a photocopied picture of my face—and jump out of the bushes with the ring, screaming, "I'm Shawn! Will you marry me?" Fortunately, I overcame the influence of my HIV meds and reconsidered that shocking scenario, opting to *really* blow her mind: I vacuumed while she was gone.

I waited for Gwenn at the airport with a "Ms. Barringer" sign. Not only that, I knew she'd be happy to return home to fresh flowers, clean carpets, and a well-hidden ring.

One of the nice things Gwenn does for me is keep my

pillbox—as well as my heart—filled. It doesn't sound like a big deal, but I appreciate that she goes to the hospital and pharmacy to get the meds for me, and somehow that gesture makes taking them a lot easier. But on this night, the pills were gone, replaced by twenty-seven little silver hearts—one for each year Gwenn has graced Earth with her presence—and one engagement ring. When she opened the compartment with a picture of her face on the front, the ring and a picture of me waited within, with the question "Will You Marry Me?"

The only hitch was that, though she noticed the pillbox immediately and found the hearts, Gwenn stopped short of opening the door with the ring. "Oh," she said, tearing up at the hearts. "That's so sweet . . . I love you." She put the pillbox aside and snuggled in with me on the couch.

"Did you see your picture?" Gwenn did. "Open that one up," I said.

She did.

She stared.

The ring sat there.

She stared some more.

The ring didn't move.

She blinked.

"What is THIS?"

Before her trip to L.A., she was a little undecided about making the cross-country flight. "No wonder you were so adamant about me going to see Jason!" I *think* she said yes, but what I remember most is telling her how Jason knew the whole time, and where I bought the ring, and how long I'd been planning this whole thing. Gwenn *loves* Clue, so part of the fun of getting *the question* was putting together the mystery of how I pulled it off.

When spring rolled around, the *Today* show announced that it was accepting online applications for the next wedding contest. The allure of worldwide fame proved to be far too intoxicating, and that night we hunched over the computer for two hours, intently studying each and every question, things like "How did you meet?" "When did you fall in love?" "Do you believe that freedom isn't free?" We finished our masterpiece and clicked the submit button, our fate now in the hands of the *Today* show.

I was still convinced that our odds were better than most, because we're camera-friendly and well-spoken. Sure, it's icy-cold silence and blank glares when no one else is around, but when Gwenn and I are in public we *shine.* If we could weasel our way into the on-air vote and make the Final Four, this thing would be an AIDS Walk.

As Gwenn and I were coiffing in the hotel room before one of our talks, the cell phone rang and I answered; it was the *Today* show! I told the producer that Gwenn *had* to be the one to get this call, would she mind calling back to surprise her when she got out of the shower?

"What's wrong with you?" Gwenn asked as I muscled my way into the bathroom.

"I need the bathroom, you've hogged it long enough!" I countered.

As we battled for the sink, the phone rang. "I'm not getting it," I said. "You jerk!" Gwenn picked up, and her expression was priceless. For twenty minutes we spoke to the producer, making jokes, telling our stories, *the works.* "You guys are *so* cute," she beamed. We were told that only about a hundred couples were getting phone calls out of a pool of about 2,500. As we finished dressing in the hotel room, we celebrated the fact that our existence of living in obscurity might be coming to an end. "Holy . . . *shit,*" Gwenn said.

It wasn't as if we were media whore novices.

Since combining our educational forces, we'd spoken to several campus newspapers, been in *Cosmopolitan* magazine, and even appeared on an MTV International special for World AIDS Day. And with celebrities frequenting the *Today* set, I knew I could hold my own with the elite of Hollywood.

At a fund-raiser for YouthAIDS hosted by Ashley Judd, Gwenn and I were presenting an award. We would be reading off of a TelePrompTer for the first time, but before we started our canned speech, I turned to Gwenn and said, into the microphone, "You know what? I think you're just as pretty as

Ashley." There were quite a few laughs, and one lady shouted, "*Just as pretty?* Gwenn is prettier!" I wondered if my mom had snuck into the building, and when discussing the outburst afterward, Gwenn told me, "That *was* Ashley Judd!"

The *Today* Show Wedding became a pageant for us, only we had no Guru to coach us and no idea whom or what we were up against. When Gwenn and I made it to the next level—the Top Ten—I was convinced we were the frontrunners. She didn't agree. "C'mon, Gwenn! They wouldn't string along a guy with AIDS, would they?" Michael and Tom concurred, and then started to argue over which of them suggested we should apply in the first place.

A small camera crew and a producer flew into Charlottesville to interview Gwenn and me at home. We needed to come up with four minutes of how we met and fell in love, and what makes our relationship unique. Well, since we speak about it all the time, we had a good forty-five minutes to whittle down. "Not so *AIDS-y*," Gwenn suggested, not wanting to scare anyone off. So our story was about triumphantly finding love and using that energy to educate others together.

After the first take, the producer looked to the camera people and said, "Do you think we need another?" They were stunned, and here's a sampling of what we laid on them: "I was diagnosed at age eleven and given two years to live. Marrying Gwenn is a dream come true, because there was a time in my life when I didn't expect to live to see this wonderful day."

Sure, it was mush. But it was good mush. *Today* show mush. If I had just sent my husband and kids off to work and school, this is the kind of mush I'd want to enjoy over a cup of coffee while waiting for *Regis & Kelly*.

Just to be safe, they filmed us a few more times, then the producer confided, "You'd be the first couple in four years that *I* would vote for."

We were supposed to hear on Thursday, and thought we were shoo-ins, until Friday rolled around and we still had not heard anything. Surely they would call us either way, right? In less than a week the Final Four videos were going to appear on television . . . Then I remembered all the great feedback we'd received up to that point and common sense took over. "We're in, Gwenn. Don't worry."

Maybe our incredible chemistry was the cause of the delay. I pictured intense negotiations going on behind the scenes about scrapping the whole dumb wedding thing and grooming these two telegenic lovebirds from Virginia to replace the on-air team of Katie Couric and Matt Lauer. I put up a good front, but I was sweating it out over the weekend, too. On Monday morning the phone rang. I let Gwenn answer so she could get the good news.

"Oh. Really?"

From the look on her face and the tone in her voice I knew we were done.

Eliminated.

Unworthy.

Forever relegated to slumming it in . . . the real world.

Playing the part of the all-American boy with AIDS now grown up got me nowhere; it was time to bring back the rebel without a cure. So, figuring that desperate times call for desperate measures, I hatched a simple plan: kidnap Al Roker.

With only two days until the Final Four couples were going to appear on the show, there was little time left to accomplish the heist. Still, it seemed doable. Al's recent gastric-bypass surgery had reduced his weight by a significant proportion, simultaneously extending his life expectancy *and* making him small enough to fit in the trunk of my car. Once Gwenn and I nabbed the lovable weatherman, we'd use Roker as a bargaining chip for a spot in the Final Four. Part of the deal, of course, would be no mention of the extortion attempt to *Today* show viewers, whom I was counting on to come through for me when *Wednesdays with Lauer* hit the shelves, just in time for Christmas.

Weirdly enough, I wasn't the only Decker contemplating a panicky last-ditch effort. When I went to the computer to e-mail everyone the bad news, I found a message from my mom, who had cc'd me on an e-mail she sent to the *Today* show:

Dear Sirs,

I just received a call from my son, Shawn Decker, that he and Gwenn Barringer did not make the final 4 couples. I am writing to ask you to reconsider 4 couples to make it 5 couples. I cannot imagine a couple more deserving than Shawn and Gwenn and ask that you reconsider. Why not let the viewers decide?

My mother, if you have not gathered, is a very passionate and protective person who has been stomping testicles since the day I was born on my behalf. She wasn't about to sit idly by and let some top-rated TV show snuff out her baby's dreams. The e-mail continued:

The only reason I can think of that they would not be chosen is AIDS. Maybe you are afraid that Gwenn might get AIDS later? Hemophiliac couples have the lowest transmission rate, nearly 0! Or maybe you are afraid of the AIDS issue. Discrimination? Or maybe a future lawsuit? What? Why? When Shawn was told he had AIDS he was only 11 and was not supposed to live a year. He never complained or cried. Today was the first time in my life that my son called me and cried.

Mom!

I couldn't believe she'd so blatantly played the "A-card." That's what my family calls it whenever I use AIDS to get out of something I don't want to do—such as a family gathering or an important test. And I *didn't* cry, even though this unceremonious rejection felt like a Pelé bicycle-kick to the nads.

To clear my good name, I sent the *Today* show the second message of the day from those ornery Deckers in Virginia.

Dear Today Show,

I apologize for my mother's spirited response to my dismissal from "Today Throws a Wedding." She's dealt with so much discrimination as a result of my HIV status: school, churches, and friends. You have to know her to understand. This whole process was quite an adventure for both Gwenn and me, and we appreciate your consideration of our application.

Shawn

P.S.: I wasn't crying. I'd just woken up.

Soon after the *Today* show dust settled, our families made it clear that their insatiable appetite for wedding cake had been whetted, and now *they* were asking the question. "So when are you two getting married?"

Now I was really angry with Couric and the Gang. Gwenn and I never planned to get married before, and now our backs were to the wall, and it was entirely their fault. But, after a few months, our opinion started to shift. "Why don't we have a wedding and do it the way *we* want it done?" No voting, no cameras, just our friends and family and a whole lot of fun. The decision was made—Gwenn and I were going to throw the ultimate party: *Weddingpalooza!*

And then my parents said the coolest thing possible: "You just let us know if you need us—and where to send the check."

Other friends chipped in, too. One offered to make the cake pro bono; musicians donated their time and skills; an artist designed the wedding invitations; and a friend who was deathly afraid of public speaking agreed to read a poem. Oh, and there was a plum spot for Katelyn, my niece. We happily employed her skills as a flower girl—and our wedding would be her fourth such gig in four years of living.

Kelly, our friend the former Baptist minister, donned his robe and performed the service admirably, sharing the duties with Virginia, a fellow case manager whom Gwenn had become close to. And Gwenn and I decided that a reception that ended at ten p.m. would never do, so we arranged for buses that would take the guests either to their hotel or to an afterparty where Bella Morte would rock out their dance-friendly goth tunes, throwing in (they promised) a crowd-pleasing cover of "Earth Angel" for the occasion. And the venue, the King Family Vineyard, which was midway between Waynesboro and Charlottesville, offered a spectacular view of the Blue Ridge Mountains. Things were coming together perfectly.

The only last-minute dash involved finding rings for the ceremony; we were stumped. Eventually we landed at a local store and met a jeweler named Biff.

Looking through the catalogue and glass display, we each found rings we really liked—and that's when Biff, who remembered a months-old newspaper article on HIV featuring a young couple, caught us off guard. "I really admire the work you two do, so I'm going to knock twenty percent off these rings." Maybe it wasn't a free wedding, but that gesture made up for *Today*'s rejection, and as we left the store, an unapologetic tear ran down my cheek.

Gwenn and I—unbeknownst to each other—had a lyric from Depeche Mode's song "Somebody" engraved on the inside of our rings. (She had "Somebody to share." I put "Somebody to love.") Another thing we agreed on was that AIDS would be banished from the wedding: no red ribbons, no tables named after HIV meds, and no mentioning of my pet virus, whom I snubbed as a groomsman.

Kip was my best man. Aside from my father and mother, I can't think of another person who's been there for me since day one—literally.

Though I'd kept my pet virus out of the wedding, I couldn't resist a tongue-in-cheek gift for my groomsmen: black-and-red letterman-style jackets with a red skull over the heart. "We're a gang now," I told them. "The Tainted Bloods."

There was no need for my new gang of pasty whiteboys to rough anyone up on our wedding day, and the weather couldn't have been better. Clouds rolled off the top of the mountain, giving an almost Nordic atmosphere to the October wedding, and it was just cool enough to keep me from sweating in my rented tux, which, thankfully, I filled out nicely. As our loved ones watched and the sun set, Gwenn

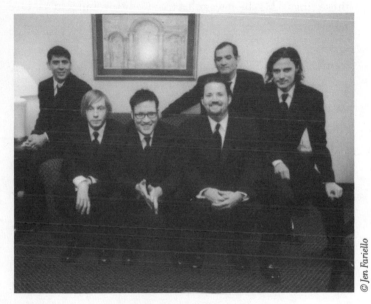

**My groomsmen and me. From left to right:
Mark, J-Woo, me, Kip, Sean, and Josh.**

and I exchanged vows we'd written for each other, and the ceremony felt so natural: in a nearby field two horses playfully "danced" with each other, as if they were celebrating the occasion. Hokey, sure, but true.

Of course, there's always the one real "moment" during every wedding, and just as poor Tom got to the middle of his spot-on poem, my great-uncle Ted started running bars on his saxophone inside the tent. Gwenn and I smiled as Kelly and Jason—Gwenn's "Best Male"—looked beseechingly out to the crowd, hoping someone would run into the tent. I'll bet Grandmother was there, looking down and laughing as her brother blew away at that sax.

Once every morsel of the delicious cake was eaten, it was off to the afterparty, where my parents arrived in rare form, dressed in leather jackets, jeans, and T-shirts that read: "Gwenn + Shawn" and "No Refunds! No Returns!"

At the end of our exhilarating (and exhausting) wedding day, Gwenn and I crashed out in each other's arms. As tired as I was, I couldn't resist asking, "Is it sexy time?"

"Hell, no," she said.

With that, we were soon asleep—in the same bed. There'd be plenty of days for sexy time in the future, and the next morning we headed home, and the only things going in our trunk were flowers, a few serving plates, and a toaster.

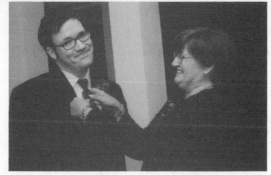

© Jen Fariello

A mother's work is never done:
fixing my tie on the wedding day.

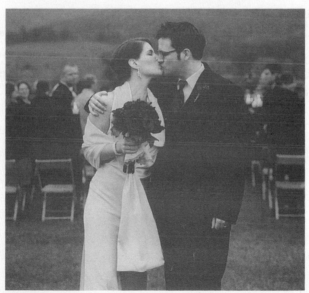

© Jen Fariello

Our wedding, 2004.

the honeymoon

A few aspects of this Saturday evening weren't out of the ordinary: it was well past midnight and I was wide awake, blogging on a computer. What was unusual was that I wasn't at home—I was in the hospital.

Five months after our wedding day, and two days before Gwenn and I were getting ready to leave for our honeymoon, I woke up at five-thirty a.m.—a sure sign of trouble. The hustle and bustle of the average workingman is something I've painstakingly avoided all my life, and the only time I do mornings is when I haven't gone to sleep yet. But this occasion wasn't by choice, and as I stood in front of the mirror, there was that old familiar feeling of blood racing down my nostril, the worst bleed since I nicked my nutsack while manscaping. I couldn't get the nosebleed to stop, so I woke Gwenn up.

"Is it bad?"

"It's bad."

"Do you think we need to go to the emergency room?"

"Yes."

Gwenn was quickly awakened by my candor; she hopped out of bed and threw on her jeans. As I stood by, ready to go while holding a reddening tissue to my nose, she grabbed the keys. "I'll drive," she said, adding, "obviously."

That afternoon I had an appointment scheduled with Dr. Greg. Two months earlier I'd gone off my HIV meds because, after close to five years on the drugs, I felt that my mind needed a break, and I really wanted to clear my head. Now it looked like I'd be arriving a little early for my one p.m. appointment with Greg.

My nose had been bleeding on and off for a couple of weeks, so I figured I was overdue for a blood-product treatment. After that I'd get lab work done, see Dr. Greg, and be back in bed in a matter of hours.

Most thinbloods would just factor up at home, but I'm pitiful; I've never self-infused, and I've been ridiculed for that in the hematology department. On a visit a few years ago I was told, "We had a six-year-old boy in here yesterday who's been treating himself for two years now!" "Oh yeah?" I said, feigning interest in the brat. In reality, I should have learned how to hit a vein. If I were ever in a real pickle, I could jab away and find something, because I know, in this case, that Gwenn would be of absolutely no help. She hates needles. And even if she learned how to do it on a piece of fruit, when the time came to actually stick me, she'd be shaking and crying, and I probably would be, too, as she closed in on me, needle in hand.

We arrived at the hospital, and soon I was whisked away to a waiting room outside the emergency room, surrounded by all of the familiar trappings of my long-forgotten childhood as a thinblood: the bed with the sheet of paper over it, the basic lifesaving equipment hanging from the walls, random charts and graphs that I've never taken the time to examine. Most people panic in this room, but my life has never hung in the balance there, and once I got my factor VIII fix I'd be good to go.

Dr. Barlada, a young resident with close-cropped hair and noticeably tattooed biceps, came walking in, kind of grunting out an awkward, monosyllabic greeting. With pen and clipboard in hand, he sat down, then asked: "How old are you? You have HIV? How long have you had it? How did you get it?"

This wasn't exactly *Murder, She Wrote*, but the guy was probably about two or three years younger than me, and it's possible that I was his first patient with hemophilia and HIV. I understand protocol—they want to make sure I'm really me—but a lot of the time, due to all the medical conditions I bring to the table, I endure a lot more gawking than most patients do.

I answered.

He grunted.

Then left.

"Gee, his bedside manner needs a little polishing," Gwenn said, breaking the tension. "Yeah," I replied, "that guy should spend a little more time on his social skills and maybe a little less time at the gym."

When Barlada returned, he was cloaked in full-on protective getup, including a face mask and plastic gloves. Universal precautions are one thing, dressing up like a character from *Star Wars* is another.

Since I had a cough, he checked my breathing, applying a cold stethoscope to my back. Then he started noodling away at one of the tray tables. I thought he was constituting the factor VIII—a simple process that includes injecting purified water into a bottle of the factor, which is a white, powdery substance that would have made a great addition to my childhood pal's fake drug bag.

Instead of a shot, Barlada clipped my nose—against my will—with two tongue depressors he'd taped together, his magic bullet for my severe nosebleed. "That should do it," he said. Shortly after he left, I took it off. Now, I've *never* yelled at someone in a hospital, and that's saying a lot, considering all of the visits I've made in my lifetime. But when Barlada

came back, not only did he ignore my explanations of hemophilia and the use of blood-product treatments, he also
threatened to write me up for refusing his state-of-the-art
"treatment."

"Get the fuck out of here, already!" I shouted.

Needless to say, Gwenn and I were far from the happiest
place on Earth.

Disney World in Orlando is where Gwenn worked for two
summers in college, and that's where we were supposed to
be going the next day for our honeymoon. But instead of
packing for our trip, Gwenn was helping to pack my bloody
nose, handing me fresh tissues.

After the dismissal of "Resident Evil," I was wheeled out
for a chest X-ray to make sure that the cough wasn't anything
serious. On the way back to the emergency room I'd set up
shop in, I saw a friendly face, a doctor from my poker night
named Buzzsaw. He was stunned to see me.

"What are you doing here?"

"Ah," I replied as I was being returned to my room. "Just
bleedin'."

After a chat with Buzz renewed my faith in the future of
medicine, a voice came over the intercom:

"Could the family of Shawn Decker come to the front desk?"

Turns out my childhood friend Photon Patrick got a
prayer chain letter on e-mail that morning that read: "Please
pray for Shawn Decker and his family. He is currently in in-
tensive care at the University of Virginia." ("Pam Decker will

not take the fall for that one!" Mom replied when I asked if she wrote it.)

When Mom arrived at the hospital, she was behaving like a Soprano, throwing her weight around, demanding answers, and even offering someone twenty dollars to get me to my own room a little faster. In her defense, I have to say that Mom has dealt with more boneheads than anyone should be subjected to, and as a result, she has no patience when it comes to dealing with less-than-competent hospital staff. It can be exhausting educating them about hemophilia, and when I was a kid I thought Mom could be unnecessarily cruel. Now, as an adult in charge of my own medical care, I realize what Mom found out years ago: Some heads need to roll.

Mom was taxed. My dad's recent scare with prostate cancer had frayed her nerves beyond repair, and now I was laid up in the hospital.

We were all worried, and soon found out what was happening: my pet virus, miffed about the wedding dis and missing his drugs, had stormed back, causing my immune system to go berserk and eat up most of my platelets, which exacerbated the nosebleed and put me at risk for internal bleeding. I got factor VIII, which did nothing, because I needed a platelet infusion, and that only worked after they put me on prednisone, a steroid.

So much for the drug holiday and the honeymoon, which

was officially off. My pet virus got his revenge, and to top it off, I had to start yet *another* new set of HIV meds.

Sean Strub researched online and was giving me updates via my cell phone as I lay in my bed, watching the news coverage of the passing of Terri Schiavo, the Florida woman in the persistent vegetative state who was taken off life support. Seeing that, I made Mom and Gwenn promise me that should things take a turn for the worse, I would be unplugged if I was still in that bed one week later. When the pope died the next day, Mom recalled the time when, as a kid, I had surgery for a hernia. "You know," she recalled, "the pope was shot the last time you spent this long in a hospital."

After three days of no sleep and the stress of wondering whether the platelet issue would be another lifelong condition, I wandered into the visitors' room, where I found an available computer, and posted a blog for my friends about plotting my escape. On Sunday morning, I informed a group of young doctors that I was going home and threw a fit when they started advising me against doing so, even though my hematologist said it would be safe. My tantrum worked: later that day, I was home in my bed.

I slept for fourteen hours.

Despite the health scare, everything was back on track rather quickly. I even resumed my promising tennis career.

Along with Bella Morte, I had formed an unofficial league called "the Children of the Court"—adorned in black leather, combat boots, and Joy Division T-shirts—that convenes on the University of Virginia's tennis courts, to the dismay of student athletes. In our league we all adopt alter egos, like pro wrestlers. I compete as the feared, behind-the-times Soviet sympathizer "Boris Decker," wearing a hammer-and-sickle T-shirt. Boris puts up a good fight, but because of a bum ankle and the fall of communism, he slows down after a couple of games.

Suddenly, though, on prednisone, instead of gimping around, I was running from side to side and tracking down shots that a few months earlier would have been difficult to reach with a ten-foot racket. My chief rival, "All-American Andy," panting after a disgraceful loss, said, "I should have you arrested for manslaughter." My victories were contested on the grounds that I was using performance-enhancing drugs, but the wins were never overturned.

Boris Decker's reign was short-lived, however, and after I was weaned off prednisone, it was back to triples play and hobbling around the court. Outside of the Children of the Court, the rest of my normal life fell into place, too. Gwenn and I were back to speaking, staying up all night watching DVDs, and enjoying last-minute board-game nights with friends. But the honeymoon . . .

It was too hot to reschedule for the summer, and that fall Gwenn and I spoke at a conference in Orlando, where we managed to slip away for a half-day to see "the Mouse," but it was hardly a substitute for a real honeymoon. Then, on our one-year wedding anniversary, we were in London. But that was part of a BBC special on AIDS—hardly a romantic outing.

You may be thinking . . . why Disney World? No, Gwenn and I aren't the fanny-pack type; and, no, we aren't going to the Magic Kingdom as a way to escape our miserable, daily existence or to celebrate a Super Bowl victory. It's fun, and it's the only place where we can tolerate children. Plus, I kind of get off on being with somebody who used to walk the grounds dressed as Pluto. Hey, don't judge.

But we're still waiting around for the perfect moment to rebook the trip. You'd think that a positoid, living with one of the most devastating medical conditions the world has seen in our lifetime, would be rushing to get to the honeymoon. Well, I've always been a procrastinator, and my pet virus hasn't influenced *all* of the decisions I've made. If that were the case, I'd be one miserable bastard.

Along the way I've discovered one thing: few people, positoid *or* negatoid, are as lucky as I am. My family rules, and I found someone who loves me enough to let me take naps—which are plentiful—whenever I need to. And I've made room in the whole deal for my pet virus. And now that it's obvious that I'm struggling down the stretch here, and the last sentences of this book are being written, I'm thinking . . . I should probably stop fucking around, and rebook that honeymoon, shouldn't I?

acknowledgments

My biggest thanks go to Gwenn for telling me to write this book—time after time—long before we'd lived many of the stories contained within. You have helped guide and protect me in so many ways, and I look forward to many more chapters with you. I love you, babe.

To Sean Strub for opening a letter ten years ago and being able to read the handwriting: thanks for the best phone call of my life. To John Berendt for giving me the confidence to start this project. To my pet agent, Christopher Schelling, for giving me a shot and making this whole book thing so enjoyable. To my editor, Ken Siman, for making this happen and believing in me and my pet virus.

Kudos to Ed Cohen, a superb copy editor, to Kevin Quirk and Paul Nolan for offering up their critical pens for initial editing, and to Erin Weed for letting me steal all of her ideas without a retaliatory judo chop to the esophagus. To Ben, my miniature-golf rival and fearless navigator of the Internet. And to The Tainted Bloods, Bella Morte, Engine Down, Lauren Hoffman, Zach, Beverly, Deanna, and Katelyn for their continued love, laughs, and devotion.

Thanks to Charlottesville—a great city full of inspiring artists—for hosting me and my pet virus.

The main obstacle in getting this book written was being alive to write it. To all the doctors, nurses, teachers, friends, and family for being on my side, even when it was the unpopular thing to do. You have earned my hugs eternally.

And lastly, to the characters who have lived *My Pet Virus* from day one: Mom, Dad, and Kip. My life was supposed to be hard, and you guys were way too easy on me. I love you for that.

ABOUT THE AUTHOR

Shawn Decker writes for *Poz* magazine and—with his "wife partner," Gwenn Barringer—travels the country, speaking candidly about sex and HIV. They live in Charlottesville, Virginia. To read his blog, visit www.mypetvirus.com.